# Praise for the first edition

*Evidence-Based Care for Normal Labour and Birth* should be a part of every midwife's library, but it should not just sit on the shelf collecting dust! It is a valuable resource and a must read for midwives, student midwives, doulas, and anyone involved in birth care.

Debra Erikson-Owen, *Journal of Midwifery & Women's Health*, USA

This scholarly, readable book provides a springboard for practitioners to jump into the deep pool of their own and their clients' experiences. It points the way toward de-medicalizing attitudes and practices around childbirth, and urges the development of a much broader range of studies and articles than now exist. Throughout, this book celebrates the dignity of childbearing women, emphasizing their need for kind, respectful, and compassionate care.

Jane Pincus, co-author of *Our Bodies, Ourselves*, USA

This book challenges midwives to look critically at their everyday practice. Not only technological interventions interfere with women's own rhythms of labour. The birth environment, the way we deal with women and the many written and unwritten rules we apply can intervene unnecessarily with the natural course of labour. This book gives you the evidence to change common practices and make them more woman-centred.

Ank de Jonge, midwife researcher, the Netherlands

As a practising midwife on a busy labour ward, I found this book brilliant for supporting and encouraging me to practice normality. Though about research in the main, it was always an interesting read with a sprinkling of anecdotes throughout the chapters. What comes through is Denis Walsh's commitment to normal birth and his passionate belief that there is a substantial amount of research out there supportive of that. I liked the broader 'take' on evidence too, not just research but clinical experience and intuition as well. Recommended for every midwife!

Labour ward midwife, Australia

As a student midwife, I have found this book great. It covers all the important research on most aspects of normal birth and the author's strong belief in the value of normal birth shines through the text. I just wish all obstetricians would read it!

Student midwife, UK

Informative and scholarly, this book is a joy to read and provides a sensible and authorative approach to the important issues of informed choice, risk and the research evidence. It will be welcomed by midwives from all areas of practice and I trust will assist them and the wider maternity care team to improve and strengthen our approach to 'best practice' in the interests of mothers and families.

Midwife teacher, UK

Denis Walsh is always such good value and a champion for normalising childbirth and seeing both sides of the 'coin'. This book leads the reader through the normal labour citing evidence to support normalising wherever possible. He offers students and midwives the opportunity to stop actively managing and consider physiologically managing what women have been doing since time began. It is written in easy text and not wrapped in waffle and academia – I thoroughly recommend.

L. Mitchell, Amazon review, UK

Far too little has been written about normality in childbirth. Denis Walsh redresses the balance and this book is essential reading for all those involved in childbirth.

Teri Gavin-Jones, UK

# Evidence and Skills for Normal Labour and Birth

Evidence-based care is a well established principle in contemporary health care and a worldwide health care movement. However, despite the emphasis on promoting evidence-based or effective care without the unnecessary use of technologies and drugs, intervention rates in childbirth continue to rise rapidly.

This new edition emphasises the importance of translating evidence into skilful practice. It updates the evidence around what works best for normal birth, aspects of which still remain hidden and ignored by some maternity care professionals. Beginning with the decision about where to have a baby, through all the phases of labour to the immediate post-birth period, it systematically details research and other evidence sources that endorse a low-intervention approach. The second edition:

- has been expanded with new chapters on preparation for childbirth and water-birth
- highlights where the evidence is compelling
- discusses its application where women question its relevance to them and where the practitioner's expertise leads them to challenge it
- gives background and context before discussing the research to date
- includes questions for reflection, skills sections and practice recommendations generated from the evidence.

Using evidence drawn from a variety of sources, *Evidence and Skills for Normal Labour and Birth* critiques institutionalised, scientifically managed birth and endorses a more humane midwifery-led model. Packed with up-to-date and relevant information, this text will help all students, practising midwives and doulas keep abreast of the evidence surrounding normal birth and ensure their practice takes full advantage of it.

**Denis Walsh** is Associate Professor in Midwifery at the University of Nottingham, UK. He lectures on evidence and skills for normal birth internationally and is widely published on midwifery issues and normal birth.

# Evidence and Skills for Normal Labour and Birth

A guide for midwives

Second edition

Denis Walsh

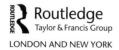
Routledge
Taylor & Francis Group

LONDON AND NEW YORK

First published in 2007
by Routledge as *Evidence-based Care for Normal Labour and Birth*

This edition published 2012
by Routledge
2 Park Square, Milton Park, Abingdon, Oxon OX14 4RN

Simultaneously published in the USA and Canada
by Routledge
711 Third Avenue, New York, NY 10017

*Routledge is an imprint of the Taylor & Francis Group, an informa business*

*British Library Cataloguing in Publication Data*
A catalogue record for this book is available from the British Library

*Library of Congress Cataloging in Publication Data*
Walsh, Denis, 1955–
Evidence and skills for normal labour and birth : guide for midwives / Denis Walsh. – 2nd ed.
 p. ; cm.
 Rev. ed. of: Evidence-based care for normal labour and birth / Denis Walsh. 2007.
 Includes bibliographical references and index.
 1. Labor (Obstetrics) 2. Childbirth. 3. Evidence-based medicine.
 I. Walsh, Denis, 1955– Evidence-based care for normal labour and birth.
 II. Title. [DNLM: 1. Natural Childbirth–nursing. 2. Evidence-Based Medicine.
 3. Midwifery. WQ 152]
 RG651.W35 2012
 618.4–dc23                                                  2011021491

ISBN: 978-0-415-57731-1 (hbk)
ISBN: 978-0-415-57732-8 (pbk)
ISBN: 978-0-203-35736-1 (ebk)

Typeset in Sabon
by Wearset Ltd, Boldon, Tyne and Wear
Printed and bound in Great Britain by
TJ International Ltd, Padstow, Cornwall

# Contents

# Foreword

*Soo Downe*

> Problems cannot be solved at the same level of awareness that created them.
>
> *Albert Einstein*

In the 1990s it seemed to many midwives in the UK that, at last, we had reached a political nirvana. The publication of *Changing Childbirth* convinced us that the social importance of good childbirth had been recognised by government bodies, excessive intervention was condemned and women's choice was accepted, lauded, even promoted above all other considerations in maternity care. For many childbirth activists, choice was supposed to lead women away from intervention, to reject epidurals and to reclaim normal birth. However, the opposite seems to be happening in many maternity units across the UK, and, indeed, across the world as a whole. In the context of increased rhetoric about the advantages of spontaneous birth, women appear to be turning towards increased technology, and, in particular, increased relief of pain in labour. What is going on?

I am increasingly of the opinion that the answer to this question lies partly with midwives. Many midwives seem to have two streams of thought running in conflict as they try to deliver the best care they can to women and babies. The first is the awareness of the need to measure, count and label labour, to fit with forms and hierarchies and systemised ways of thinking. The second is the subtle narrative that many practitioners hear during childbirth. It could be called intuition, or expertise, or empathy, or any number of things – but what it is is the continually updated message that records and flexes around an individual labour – the recognition of 'unique normality' which Robbie Davis-Floyd and Elizabeth Davis first discussed.[1] The real problem for many midwives in hectic, sometimes impossibly busy clinical practice is how to hear and act on this second voice.

Our beliefs about childbirth are the fundamental base on which we interpret and build 'evidence'. Midwifery knowledge at its best recognises unique normality, responds ahead of absolute emergencies, constantly assesses the complex situation of a birth, pregnancy or postnatal episode, and constantly factors in the woman herself, her family culture and her particular philosophies, ideals, hopes and aspirations, as well as the formal evidence base. This approach to midwifery knowledge makes no assumptions about the inevitability of any occurrence, but keeps all possible events in a subtle background mental balance with an informed intuition and empathetic awareness. Coming to birth with this mind-set recognises that birth is complex and individual, and allows each birth to add new knowledge.

In this balanced, practical and insightful book, Denis Walsh has managed the extraordinary feat of providing an insight into how this kind of midwifery works. By exploring the practical implications of seeing labour as a process of rhythms rather than of phases, contextualised by the relevant historical, philosophical, theoretical and evidential literature, he offers the possibility of legitimately reframing what birth is, and what it could be. He notes that, although there is little authoritative evidence in this area, there is a large and increasing body of knowledge that is not being put into practice. It is this knowledge that he is offering for our consideration. In addition, and crucially, he also proposes ways of moving forward on the basis of this approach that can be implemented in any setting.

His technique of effectively integrating narrative and evidence, and of subverting usual ways of thinking, provides readers of this book with the tools to move to a new level of awareness, and therefore with an effective response to Einstein's challenge in the quotation above. The potential for positive responses to the current problems in midwifery practice and maternity care across the world is enormous, and I look forward to seeing what happens next...

Professor Soo Downe
University of Central Lancashire

## Note

1 Davis-Floyd, R. and Davis, E. (1997) Intuition as authoritative knowledge in midwifery and home birth. In R. Davis-Floyd and P.S. Arvidson (eds) *Intuition: The Inside Story – Interdisciplinary Perspectives*. New York: Routledge.

# Foreword

*Sheila Kitzinger*

In this exciting book, Professor Walsh questions interventions carried out by both obstetricians and midwives that research evidence now reveals can be iatrogenic. Women have been brainwashed into believing that if management protocols for practices such as routine induction, if a pregnancy exceeds the time allotted to it by professional managers, and drugs to rev up the labour, when a cervix does not dilate by at least 1 cm an hour, are not administered, then their babies will suffer and be brain damaged or die. Many practices in managing labour may appear innocuous but lead to instrumental delivery, caesarean section and, in turn, to intense pain, opiates and epidurals, haemorrhage and blood clots. Women should know this if they are to make informed choices and, perhaps even more important, informed refusals.

In this new edition, Denis Walsh sketches the development of antenatal education, tracing it back to Grantly Dick-Read. In the five years before the publication of my first book, *The Experience of Childbirth*, in 1962 (1) I had been running antenatal classes for the NCT based on much of what Dick-Read taught. My method also drew on the Stanislavsky school of acting and techniques of using touch and emotion memory to help relaxation. Arne Jacobson was the first to draw attention to the relationship between fear and pain in 1930. Grantly Dick-Read, who was working in South Africa, also drew from Dr Kathleen Vaughan, who had observed women squatting in childbirth when she was in India, and the obstetric physiotherapist Helen Herdman.

Accouchement sans douleur, or ASD, brought in ideas from Russia based on Pavlovian psychology and research with salivating dogs and experiments with conditioned reflexes to raise the pain threshold. Women used breathing techniques involving distraction, 'huff and puff', 'slump and blow', 'choo-choo' and 'the sigh', along with breathing levels A, B, C and D. A woman had to perform well with these or she had failed. Lamaze in Paris claimed that over 18 per cent succeeded completely and just over 4 per cent failed (2). French psychoprophylaxis urged women to put on a star performance.

Psychoprophylaxis in Russia, France and the USA was a complete contrast to Dick-Read's teaching. It called relaxation by a new name – 'decontraction'. As the system spread, breathing exercises proliferated. Wherever antenatal classes were taught there seemed to be some new variation or complication of exercises. On lecture tours across the USA, Canada and the UK, I was often asked if I myself taught 'tune-tapping', 'H out', 'whoo' or 'ssssss'. It all tended to be very noisy and labour wards hummed with activity as women tried to pant like a dog through contractions, often to the consternation and dismay of midwives. Dissociation was the main theme for all these exercises, with the idea that the woman would concentrate on some activity so hard that she was distracted from pain. She was taught how to block pain sensations, and failed at the first real pain.

The Natural Childbirth Society was formed in the 1960s by Prunella Briance, a passionate believer in Dick-Read's teaching, and it was when what became the National Childbirth Trust rejected her leadership that psychoprophylaxis took over from the Dick-Read approach.

In this edition there is also a new chapter on immersion in water for labour and, if women choose this, waterbirth. The use of a birth pool arose out of a concern to give babies a positive transition to life, and even before that, to make them healthy and vigorous. That, too, started in Russia with Igor Charkovsky, a boat builder, who, in the role of shaman, threw babies into the Black Sea, or, failing that, into a large pool filled with iced water, to toughen them up. It was nothing to do with the gentleness that we now associate with waterbirth and loving care of the newborn. Charkovsky came to conduct a workshop in my house and I felt the need to stop him on entry, telling him that under no circumstances could he throw a baby into the pool that he had ordered to be set up. He didn't. But he demonstrated how to 'straighten the spine' by extending and twisting it, seizing a baby as she was suckling at her mother's breast and screwing her round. He was concerned to 'break the barrier of pain' and produce a child able to take on the challenges of life.

Frederic LeBoyer studied what was happening in Russia and created his own very different version of helping babies to adapt to life, with tenderness and joy. He was not talking about the mother. She gave birth on land. But the baby was lifted into water afterwards.

Then Michel Odent, not an obstetrician but a surgeon who questioned why he was doing so many caesareans at his clinic in Pithiviers, gave women the opportunity to labour and give birth in water. The first time a baby was born under water he was surprised and quickly stepped in to deliver it – still wearing his socks. I worked with several colleagues in the birth movement to invite him over to the UK to describe his approach. That was the start of waterbirth here. My first grandson was born in a pool in my home – only the second waterbirth in this country. He did not cry. His mother lifted him up and he looked in her eyes and smiled. Like Denis Walsh, I know at first hand how beautiful waterbirth can be (3).

Walsh explores the reasons why midwives may discourage use of a pool – because it takes more one-to-one time with a woman than standard birth practices, and diverts midwives from caring for patients who have had an epidural – and describes the strategies they adopt to refuse women the chance to labour in water. This analysis is an important addition to the literature on what are considered 'alternative practices'.

I believe that this book will be of great help to students and practising midwives, and open the way to deeper awareness of their role in helping women in childbirth with quiet, continuous, personal support without directing, dogmatising, yelling 'Push!' or other potentially harmful interventions.

Today there is a new political awareness not only among birth activists but among midwives and many obstetricians. I believe that acknowledgement of the politics of midwifery is a basic condition for change. Midwives need to develop a co-ordinated, flexible strategy working across the globe with childbearing women. To do this we need a wider perspective and a historical sense. Since the Middle Ages there has been a concerted effort, first from the Church and then from the medical system, to destroy midwifery as a female vocation with its own standards. The medical system has derided, discredited, humiliated and threatened midwives, and attempted to reduce them to the status of domestic servants. This book points the way to the future.

Sheila Kitzinger
www.sheilakitzinger.com

# Preface

Four years have passed since this book was first published. Over that period I have had feedback from midwives, student midwives, doulas, antenatal education teachers and birthing women from all over the world about how it has encouraged them to pursue their ideal of supporting and achieving low-intervention, physiological birth. One email that sticks in my mind arrived in the wake of the controversy in 2009 over comments in the press I had made concerning labour pain, where I was largely misquoted and misrepresented. It said:

> I don't believe the same person that wrote *Evidence-Based Care for Normal Labour and Birth* would have said the things reported in the press regarding women and labour pain. The former I recognise as a keen observer and practitioner of birth, the latter seems a detached academic with an axe to grind.

I cherished that email among a barrage of largely negative feedback.

Two years on from that experience it is time to update this text. New evidence is arriving all the time, mostly supportive of normal labour and birth, though arguments still rage about place of birth and the appropriateness of drug-free birth. The context in which childbirth occurs has moved on since 2007, with a much greater awareness now of the spectre of maternal and perinatal mortality in the developing world. Alongside that change, the ubiquity of risk in Western maternity care systems continues to impact on practice. Economic rationalism is also continuing to drive change in provision with the increasing centralisation of birthing. This presents opportunities for midwifery-led care to establish low-tech alternative birth environments, shored up by the recent positive systematic review of midwifery-led care in the Cochrane Database (Hatem *et al.* 2008).

Midwifery research has also grown since 2007, with new journals coming on stream showcasing the increasing body of midwifery-led research. *Women and Birth* from Australia and the *International Journal of Childbirth* are two new titles.

This edition has been expanded to cover omissions from the first edition and has new chapters on 'Preparation for childbirth' and 'Water immersion and waterbirth'. In addition, all other chapters have been updated with current evidence. The other change from the first edition is the expansion of evidence to include skills; hence the new title *Evidence and Skills for Normal Labour and Birth*. My approach to skills here is not to cover generic technical and procedural skills that are available in a number of other texts, but to examine skill as decision-making against a background of uncertainty. I also share practical tips that have surfaced during the Enhancing Skills for Normal Labour and Birth course that I have been running over the past two years.

Denis Walsh
Nottingham University
United Kingdom, 2011

# Acknowledgements

I want to pay tribute to all the midwives I have had the privilege to meet in many different places, who are quietly and courageously fleshing out the evidence presented in this book in challenging circumstances. They are working mostly in consultant maternity hospitals that are generally more focused on obstetric priorities and management-led, short-term financial targets than an agenda around normal birth. In these challenging circumstances they continue to fly the flag for optimising birth physiology.

Also to my academic and clinical colleagues from a number of universities and maternity services around the world, who are inspiring in their commitment to normal birth and pioneering in their research in this crucial area of women's health. I would especially like to mention the now annual International Normal Birth Conference that takes place across the globe in different continents but which originated in the UK under the tutelage of Soo Downe. I would urge every midwife to attend this conference once in their professional life. It is an awe-inspiring event that will reinforce or reconnect you with a vision for normal birth in the twenty-first century.

Thank you also to Kate Evans, author of *The Food of Love*, for her illustrations.

# Chapter 1    Knowledge, evidence and skills for normal birth

- Critiques of the evidence paradigm
- Qualitative research
- Models and underpinning tenets of childbirth care
- Skills and evidence
- Conclusion
- Questions for reflection

Evidence-based care has bedded down as a mainstream paradigm in health care over the last five years. Within the UK, the National Institute for Clinical Excellence (NICE) continues to issue national guidelines on a plethora of areas of health care, predicated on a robust methodology of appraising and integrating the best available evidence. Guidelines for practice have become commonplace and normative in maternity provider settings. In fact, they have become even more authoritative because providers' safety and quality agendas are underpinned by such guidelines. How clinical guidelines feed into levels of indemnity insurance cover for the Clinical Negligence Scheme for Trusts (CNST) which operates in England and Wales is a good example.

Yet, concerns remain about the politics of evidence: how it is distilled at a national level (Milewa and Barry 2005), how it is enacted at a local level (Nettleton et al. 2008) and how individual practitioners interpret and apply it (Kulier et al. 2008). Rogers (2004) problematises evidence-based medicine in relation to women's health, arguing that gender bias affects both the choice of research topics (a focus on technology and pathology) and the methods chosen to research, analyse and synthesise them (randomised controlled trials (RCTs) and statistical analysis over lived experience), as well as guideline development (under-representation of women and consumers).

Earlier, Pope (2003) had traced the evidence paradigm's epidemiological roots, characterising it as a social movement whose spread in Western health care has been remarkable since the mid-1990s. Large sections of the health professions, health care managers and finally governments themselves have embraced it with an almost evangelical fervour. Rather simplistic slogans have trumpeted its common-sense appeal. 'Doing the right thing, in the right way at the right time to the right patient' was one nursing rendition of its intent (RCN 1998). Others have simply stated that it is about doing what works, what is effective.

## Critiques of the evidence paradigm

Critics' objections, noted above (Nettleton et al. 2008, Kulier et al. 2008), were to do with the contingent nature of clinical practice and the professional's role in exercising clinical judgement with their patients, many of whom were not the typical 'average' patient identified in research studies. Both surgeons and physicians claimed that clinical decision-making was an art as well as a science and that intuitive judgements and 'hunches' were as much a part of the armoury for clinical decision-making as research knowledge.

Sackett's (1996) original paper on evidence-based medicine (EBM) was actually explicit about the role of experience/expertise in contributing to evidence-based decision-making, as well as another variable: patient's preferences.

Measuring fixed clinical outcomes is insufficient when studying human beings. The research participant's subjective experience of the intervention or treatment must also be examined, as should its impact on significant others. The Cochrane Database is full of trials where these elements were omitted, though this is changing. Enkin *et al.* (2000), writing at the time of the first publication of the Cochrane Database, made an intriguing comment on the limitations of quantitative enquiry when he said: 'sometimes, what really counts, cannot be counted.' He was acknowledging the profundity of the childbirth experience, which, in terms of its effects, cannot be reduced to simple statistics.

Another weakness in quantitative research is its assumption, already alluded to, that population studies are directly applicable to individuals. Evidence-based guidelines are premised on this assumption, underpinned as they are by the most robust research evidence available. By their very nature, clinical trials are selective of their samples and attempt to control for variables that could introduce bias. In other words, the research process is 'hot-housed' in an effort to distil the purest findings. But this very process makes generalisability problematic because the real world of practice does not operate in such a sanitised way. An interesting example of this recently occurred on a delivery suite where a woman came in to labour, having had twelve babies before. The protocol, based on studies that concluded there was a link between high parity and third-stage haemorrhage, required her to have a venflon inserted and an intravenous infusion of oxytocin with the third stage of labour. She disagreed with this, stating that there had never been problems with the third stage of labour before. She challenged the findings of population-based studies by stating that her body was different from this statistical norm.

A further area where the evidence dogma is vulnerable is deciding what to do when the research results are equivocal in a clinical area or research has simply not been done. To address the area of the robustness of different quantitative research designs, hierarchy of evidence tables have been developed that guide clinicians in appraising the strength of evidence. This list also helps them when confronted with no research or uncertain research results. A consensus of clinical experts should guide practice when research is absent. But this statement begs the question: which experts? Miller and Petrie (2000) call this method GOBSAT (good old boys sat at table), listing the various biases that the method is likely to lead to. Evidence hierarchies are useful for comparing different quantitative methods but what if these methods don't suit the situation under scrutiny? Increasingly, health care professionals are seeing the limitations of reductionist research methods when dealing with complex interventions. In maternity care, models of midwifery care fall into this category, and RCTs have limited utility when evaluating all the nuances of continuity of care, midwifery-led care, caseload models and birth centre care. As Downe and McCourt (2008) rightly point out, quantitative research is predicated on the attainment of certainty, the principle of linearity (cause and effect can be discretely linked) and simplicity. They suggest that this is a poor fit with contemporary health care, which has few certain outcomes, multi-factorial causation and effects and is best understood as a complex system.

Over the last three years, there has been a proliferation of clinical guidelines, emanating from national bodies like NICE that are increasingly regulating practice. It is hard to argue against their efficacy, especially when based on the best available research, but social science researchers have challenged their 'neutral' status (Hunter and Segrott 2008). Clinical guidelines are social constructions as well as clinical templates that have a range of impacts including constructing decision-making as a linear process, standardising practices (one size fits all) and prescribing documentation (Berg 1997). Tentative evidence suggests that clinical guidelines may be helpful for the novice but constricting for the expert (Greatbatch *et al.* 2005), though both as employees are accountable to employer directives. As reflective autonomous practitioners, we have a responsibility and a prerogative to make the best clinical judgements we can in partnership with women, even if this means going against normative practice.

## Qualitative research

There is increasing recognition that qualitative research has an important role to play in addressing the complexities of practice. In fact, much of the problematising of the evidence paradigm has arisen from qualitative investigation, as Hunter and Segrott's (2008) review illustrates. Qualitative research has the power to explain multi-layered phenomena. My interest in qualitative research goes back to the late 1980s when I first read Kirkham's (1989) study of communication in labour. I could not believe how she was able to describe so accurately the clinical environment I was working in. Not only could she reflect back to me what I was seeing every day, but she was able to conceptualise it in a novel way. Her explanation of the journey from independent woman to passive patient helped me see hospital labour ward care through new eyes. She articulated its institutionalising and disempowering effects. I knew there were things wrong with the way care was delivered, but she explained it in a fresh way. It was like 'the penny dropping' or a 'light going on', and I now had a better understanding of what was wrong with hospital birth. Qualitative research seemed to achieve something that years of looking at quantitative research had never achieved: a new way of seeing things. It was subsequently perplexing for me to read that critics of qualitative research believed it did not constitute evidence because it was not generalisable beyond the immediate environment it described.

Even acknowledging that qualitative research and clinical experience play important parts in a broader understanding of evidence, there may be other sources of 'knowing' that can illuminate our understanding. Common sense tells us that some things work better than others and there is no need to run an RCT on the obvious. I wonder whether we have reached that point in researching relational aspects of care, specifically comparing fragmented models of labour provision with models that offer known carers. Surely the vast majority of women, if given a choice between carers known to them and strangers, would choose the former as their labour guides. In the chapter on first-stage labour rhythms (Chapter 4), I will apply this critique to the vexed question of the best model of early labour care, which has been a target for researchers over the past three years. The tentative conclusion: attendance at home by a carer you know already is the best model.

Having worked in midwifery-led units and talked to many midwives in these settings, my own view is that midwives also learn and add to their knowledge base through what Polanyi (1994) calls 'personal knowledge'. In the best paper on this type of knowing, Gabbay and le May's (2004) research in GPs' decision-making describes how this knowledge is attained through doing, reflecting and sharing with colleagues in similar situations – what they call 'mindlines'. These are collectively reinforced, internalised, tacit guidelines that practitioners apply through learning in praxis. There is a considerable body of writing within nursing, drawing on Benner's (1984) novice-to-expert trajectory, Schon's (1995) knowing in action, Johns' (1995) reflective practice and Carper's (1978) stages of knowing, that supports 'personal knowledge' as a major contributor to evidence in practice.

So far evidence has been sourced to research both quantitative and qualitative, clinical experience, women's preferences, common sense and personal knowing through thinking about practice. Childbirth has been around a long time and therefore it also may be fruitful to examine anthropological sources for evidence. Birth posture is a good example. Archaeological 'evidence' from thousands of years ago (Egyptian, Roman and Greek civilisations) and anthropological 'evidence' from indigenous tribal groups across the planet today support the idea that the adoption of upright posture for birth has been common for human beings for millennia. The majority of the research studies are no more than thirty years old, with principal RCTs more recent than that. Are we really saying in our Western arrogance that we have nothing to learn from these sources?

Fry's excellent paper (2007a) groups all midwifery knowledge sources noted above under the umbrella heading of intuition. In doing so, she gives space for the wise combination of the art and science of midwifery in clinical practice. Intuition has been given a range of meanings in the literature (Davis-Floyd and Davis 1997), which includes the more populist notion of a sudden hunch, but feminist writings have challenged us to consider its application in the context of connection and 'sussing out' (LoCicero 1993). LoCicero argues that caesarean rates might come down if obstetricians and midwives intuit care scenarios better by connecting and listening to women, rather than standing outside a situation of uncertainty to evaluate it objectively. Parratt and Fahy (2008) make a similar point in their plea to incorporate the non-rational into midwifery decision-making. Intuition, for Fry, covers all these contingencies of knowledge for practice and her paper attempts to rehabilitate a word that is highly regarded by midwives and women, yet undervalued and marginalised within the conventional evidence paradigm.

All of these reflections indicate to us that evidence is not a neutral concept – it is politically laden, with various interest groups standing to gain or lose from the adoption of their particular 'take' on evidence. Stewart (2001) and Milewa and Barry (2005) have discussed this dimension. Therefore for the purpose of this book, I want to be explicit about the values and beliefs underpinning the concept here. My 'take' on evidence endorses the two principles that Enkin *et al.* (2000) enunciated in the late 1980s when the Cochrane Database was first published. Their principles are paraphrased here:

- Don't intervene in physiology unless the intervention is known to be more effective than nature.
- Ensure the intervention has no side-effects that outweigh the benefit.

## Models and underpinning tenets of childbirth care

Enkin *et al.* had an acute sensitivity to the ancient Hippocratic injunction – 'First, do no harm' – and recognised the dangers of iatrogenesis. The onus is clearly on the person introducing an intervention to prove its superiority over what is happening naturally. In other words, it is a position of humility before the physiology that respects it, believes in it and affirms it unless pathology manifests. If childbirth professionals had adopted this position, we would not have set about 'managing' labour and birth as though it cannot be trusted.

The management approach is indicative of the values and beliefs underpinning the biomedical model and in this chapter I want to predicate the understanding of evidence not on a biomedical model of childbirth but in a social model (Walsh and Newburn 2002). Table 1.1 contrasts these two approaches.

Since 2007, rhetoric has softened in academic journals on the dichotomising of models of care because it is recognised that a large degree of overlap occurs between biomedical and social models of health (Van Teijlingen 2005). For example, institutional birth settings are engaging now with the imperative to humanise the birth space (Fannon 2003) and few would now sustain a position that all obstetricians subscribe fully to a biomedical ethos or that all midwives embrace a social model of care. Nevertheless, illustrating contrasting beliefs in a table is still a useful heuristic device to prompt discussion and debate.

I would add to the values of a social model by explicitly stating my profound belief in midwifery-led care and midwifery autonomy in normal labour and birth care. The midwife should be the lead carer for physiological childbirth. Within this dynamic she should seek to work in partnership with women, premising her care on the key themes of choice, continuity and control.

Any discussion of evidence needs to engage with women's priorities and, in general terms, these can be summarised from the extensive evaluative and survey literature of recent decades. The three Cs (continuity, choice, control) come from these sources and are official maternity care policy in many countries. Information is a fourth theme that is implicit in good maternity care policy. Since the early 1990s, research has been better able to tease out the layers of meaning behind these themes that all multi-disciplinary maternity groups have enthusiastically signed up to. The phrases have been in danger of becoming empty rhetoric as various stakeholders have interpreted them

TABLE 1.1

| Social model | Biomedical model |
| --- | --- |
| Whole person – physiology, psychosocial, spiritual | Reductionism – powers, passages, passenger |
| Respect and empower | Control and manage |
| Relational/subjective | Expertise/objective |
| Environment central | Environment peripheral |
| Anticipate normality | Anticipate pathology |
| Technology as servant | Technology as partner |
| Celebrate difference | Homogenisation |
| Intuition/meaning-making | Quantitative research/objective facts |
| Self-actualisation | Safety |

pragmatically, hedging them around with restrictions due to local conditions. The limiting of the home birth option and the winding down of continuity schemes are two examples.

Green and colleagues' seminal study, *Great Expectations* (1998), clearly showed that all groups of women want information and that clinicians should not withhold information according to the social class or ethnic background of women. Less well known from their work is the role of expectations in shaping childbirth experience. They found that women who approach labour and birth with an optimistic mindset did better than women who had a more fearful, negative attitude. It pointed to the exciting possibility that midwives had a window of opportunity antenatally to examine and gently challenge negative and anxious dispositions to see if women could adopt a more positive outlook.

Informed choice has been examined in some depth by researchers, and Kirkham's (2004) excellent edited book thoroughly discusses the various nuances of the concept. Among a number of insights, they highlight how choices can be limited by providers and that deprivation and other con-straints may restrict women's access to those choices that are available. Women tell stories of not being offered home or birth centre options when booking for care, or being unable to afford to travel to a birth centre which may be some distance away. Informed choice is not a level playing field for all women. Levy (1999) has shown how the framing of information pro-foundly shapes choice in her study of midwives' encounters with women in antenatal clinics. She coined the phrase 'gently steering' to capture the dynamic of how midwives coax women to choices that the midwives are comfortable with. A much more worrying dynamic is the blackmail approach to influencing choice where, in response to the question 'What would you recommend?', the professional's response is: 'Well, if you were my partner, I would say...'

In a similar way, 'control' has been deconstructed to show a number of interpretations. Most maternity care providers probably understand control as women's ability to retain control over decision-making during labour but research has revealed that, for many women, control is understood as control over their body's response to the awesome power of labour or retaining psy-chological control during labour while their body feels out of control (Green 1999). Other researchers have highlighted the paradox of women retaining control by giving up their bodies to the professionals to be managed by them (Zadoroznyi 1999). It seems that a fear of the labour and birth events some-times drives this and highlights the fact that evidence in the contemporary childbirth context has to be understood against a background of increasing medicalisation.

Tracey *et al.* (2007), Mead (2008) and Declerq *et al.* (2002) paint a picture of a widespread collapse of confidence among low-risk women, in particular, in an ability to do birth without routine intervention. Their Australia-, UK- and USA-based studies reveal alarming intervention rates in this group, with as little as 17 per cent labouring and birthing physiologically. Other countries are documenting the rise of tocophobia (morbid fear of labour) in another manifestation of this crisis (Laursen *et al.* 2008).

This takes us back to one of the purposes behind this book – to highlight the extensive body of research that supports the physiology of labour and birth. This body of work is obscured by the dominant focus in medical journals and in local service provision on childbirth pathologies and the technologies that treat them. It leads to the undervaluing and under-investment in midwifery-mediated care, though it is known to be efficacious (Hatem *et al.* 2008). Another purpose is to examine other factors that optimise both the physiology and the experience of childbirth for our generation of women. This focus is on birth environment, relational components of care and the role of personal birth philosophy in maximising well-being or 'salutogenesis' (Downe and McCourt 2008).

Finally, we are working with evidence sources, especially in relation to research, that are circumscribed by the setting in which the vast majority of inquiry was carried out. And that is not just hospitals but very large hospitals. We must ask the question: does all this research tell us about physiological birth or about how women's bodies behave when observed in a hospital setting? We won't be able to fully answer that question until the studies have been done in and out of hospital birth settings. In the meantime, we work with what we have, but our critical faculties will reserve a comprehensive judgement.

The setting for birth also brings into play organisational factors that impinge on evidence. With the trend towards increasingly large institutions for birth, we have to engage with the particular pressures this brings to the childbirth event. Some of these are temporal (to do with time pressures), some institutional (to do with constraints and regulation) and some bureaucratic (to do with power differentials within professional groups and between professionals and women). I therefore preface the discussion of evidence over the coming chapters with an alignment to small scale as an optimum model of organisation, and would juxtapose two models as shown in Table 1.2.

We now know that the context of practice impinges heavily on decisions with evidence that the same midwives will make different clinical decisions depending on whether they are attending a home birth, birth in a midwifery-led unit (MLU) or birth on a labour ward (Crabtree 2008). For a more in-depth discussion of the implications of these contrasting organisational

TABLE 1.2

| Large scale | Small scale |
| --- | --- |
| Bureaucratic | Pragmatic |
| Institutional | Homely |
| Hierarchical | Non-hierarchical |
| Impersonal | Personal |
| Formal | Informal |
| Rigidity | Flexibility |
| Standardised | Individualised |
| Control | Autonomy |
| Throughput | Input |
| Risk | Efficacy |
| Organisation | Community |
| Time-bound | 'Go with the flow' |
| 'Doing' | 'Being' |

models, drawing on research into a free-standing birth centre, I would recommend my paper in *Social Science & Medicine* (Walsh 2006b).

Finally, the concept of embodiment has at last attracted midwifery interest as it is central to how practitioners and women approach the body in birth. Attitudes to the body have been the subject of sociological inquiry for many years but writing on childbirth embodiment has been notably absent from these discussions until recently. Davis and Walker (2010) have brought the natural body and the socially constructed body theories to our attention, demonstrating how they have influenced the medicalisation of birth and the natural childbirth movement over recent decades. I have added my own reflections to theirs (Walsh 2010), restating the neglected theory of the 'lived' or 'phenomenological' body in birth. This attempts to rehabilitate women's autonomy and agency over their own body in birth, as it is subjected to practitioner and institutional 'takes' on what birthing is like or how it should be done. The lens of embodiment filters evidence in subtle but powerful ways and an awareness of the concept is therefore important.

## Skills and evidence

The utilisation of evidence in practice is clearly not just about head knowledge. The translation into practice requires considered decision-making, often against a background of uncertainty, and then the engagement of skills. Since 2007, I have changed the focus of the evidence course to concentrate more on using evidence in practice to address this need. Sometimes the application of evidence requires nuanced decision-making (diagnosing delay in labour), sometimes practical skills (assisting a physiological third stage), sometimes psychological skills (assisting a woman through labour pain), sometimes technical skills (interpreting a CTG) and sometimes procedural skills (urinary catheterisation). I am not addressing technical or procedural skills here as there are excellent texts on these already. It is the first three that I will refer to in subsequent chapters.

Somewhat surprisingly, there is not a lot of research into midwifery decision-making (Jefford *et al.* 2010). What there is reveals an interesting web of overlapping factors such as the setting (Crabtree 2008), the perception of risk (Lankshear *et al.* 2005), professional paternalism (de Jonge *et al.* 2008) and bureaucratic and rule-based approaches (Porter *et al.* 2007). As Porter and colleagues comment, in spite of midwifery's woman-centred ethos, there is little empirical evidence of a shared decision-making model in practice, except in the caseload midwifery literature (Finlay and Sandall 2009).

The nature of decision-making is that it is dynamic and contextual and therefore difficult to capture in the one-dimensional frame of writing on a page, as opposed to interactive discussion with individuals reviewing their real experiences. However, case scenarios will be presented in some chapters in an attempt to prompt reflection.

Paradoxically, practical skills for supporting normal birth can be as much about unlearning, 'sitting on one's hands' and literally doing nothing. Accompanying upright birth positions, assisting a physiological third stage and attending a waterbirth may mean doing less rather than doing more. Yet there is a skill to 'masterly inactivity', as the Royal College of Midwives' Campaign for Normal Birth states. Their website quotes an ancient Chinese sage, Lao Tzu, who said: 'The perfect practitioner appears to do nothing, yet nothing is left undone' (www.rcmnormalbirth.org.uk/stories/on-the-crest-of-a-wave/masterly-inactivity).

Clearly there is overlap between practical and psychological skills, with the latter showing itself most potently in supporting women through labour pain. Read Leap *et al.*'s (2010) instructive paper on the power of relational continuity in this context, which will be returned to in the chapter on pain and labour (Chapter 7).

## Conclusion

Evidence-based care has been around long enough now to have passed through a 'honeymoon period', a resistance phase and a critical appraisal, so it has 'matured' as a concept. From its original orthodoxy emphasising the research base of a variety of interventions, there is a substantial body of evidence around normal birth that is now 'available' for implementation. Maternity service providers are beginning to structure care to maximise the utilisation of this body of evidence. Within the UK, services are being performance managed on providing a midwifery-led care pathway that includes intrapartum provision (Department of Health 2008), and in Australia, midwifery-led care is beginning to be enshrined in statute (Report of the Maternity Services Review 2009). At last services are starting to view existing normal birth research as a lifeline to the maternity services struggling with the challenge of medicalisation, the spiralling cost of high-tech maternity care, the 'how' of addressing the quality and safety agenda and issues around the recruitment and retention of midwives.

But the really exciting dimension of a broader understanding of evidence is its potential to rehabilitate physiological birth as not only possible, but desirable for the vast majority of this generation of women. Evidence that springs from intuitive, experiential and anthropological origins as well as research has the power to reconnect us to the transformative nature of this ancient rite-of-passage event. And then not only individual women but families, communities and even nations will benefit.

## Questions for reflection

How would you define evidence-based care?

Can you think of examples where you used intuition or common sense to guide clinical decision-making?

What role should qualitative research play in evidence-based care?

Do organisational pressures impact on evidence-based decision-making? How?

Where do you sit on the continuum between a biomedical and a social model of childbirth?

What is your own view of the body in birth (embodiment)? Does it influence how you practise?

# Chapter 2 **Preparation for childbirth**

- A brief history of models and approaches
- Focus of educational content and evidence base
- Specific therapies and new approaches to antenatal care provision
- New directions and conclusion
- Practice recommendations
- Questions for reflection

Green and Baston's (2007) research into the changing expectations of child-bearing women, which showed their increasing openness to routine labour interventions like induction of labour and epidurals in particular, is challenging for maternity services. Globally, makers of maternity service policy have become concerned about increased rates of intervention, as have midwives. The challenge arises when users of the service don't necessarily share this concern. Within a climate of informed choice, it is hard to see how a low-intervention birth can be promoted when women enter the maternity services already favourably disposed to drugs and technology.

Several decades ago it was recognised that education during pregnancy, focused on childbirth and early parenting, may be beneficial to women who enter the maternity services with vastly contrasting knowledge bases and prior experience. Since that time a variety of models of childbirth education have evolved. Contemporary childbirth education is morphing again in response to the changing needs of women, but, for midwives, this issue of how to challenge the increasingly biomedical focus that emanates from women themselves is a particular priority. In this chapter, the recent history and approaches used in childbirth education will be summarised and its evidence base appraised. In the past three years, newer approaches with an emerging evidence base have been trialled. These will be examined in more detail to see what lessons can be gleaned for midwives who, in the majority of cases, facilitate and provide this type of education. Finally, I will make some reflections about future priorities and directions.

## A brief history of models and approaches

Education for childbirth programmes began in the USA in the 1960s and have spread throughout the Western world since then (Walker *et al.* 2009). The rationale for their introduction was based on women's inhumane treatment in maternity hospitals and concerns even back then that too many drugs were routinely being given during labour. Women needed to be armed with information that would help them negotiate their way through labour in this suboptimal environment. One key aspect of this was the management of pain.

Over the next twenty years, different approaches evolved to address this particular area. In the USA, the Lamaze and Bradley methods dominated, while in the UK, psychoprophylaxis (a variant of Lamaze), the Active Birth Movement and the National Childbirth Trust decisively influenced NHS hospital provision through to 2000 and beyond.

The grandfather of all these approaches was arguably Grantly Dick-Read, whose seminal text *Childbirth without Fear* can still be purchased today.

Dick-Read's idea that ignorance of what to expect in labour is likely to rein-force fear, setting up a fear–pain–fear cycle, was validated in part seventy years later by Lang *et al.*'s (2006) research demonstrating that anxiety pre-dicts labour pain. Rather controversially, Dick-Read advocated that it was possible to experience a pain-free birth if anxiety was taken away and, again decades later, the hypno-birthing movement has reprised this idea (Mongan 2005).

However, the initial impetus of *Childbirth without Fear* was capitalised on by the French obstetrician Fernand Lamaze, who introduced and promoted a package to pregnant women combining childbirth education, relaxation and breathing techniques. Others developed his package, coining the term 'psy-choprophylaxis' as a descriptor of the Lamaze method and promoted it throughout the USA. The original emphases on controlled breathing and progressive relaxation techniques have given way to an explicit philosophy supporting normal labour and birth. Today the organisation promotes six care practices to optimise normal birth (see Box 2.1).

---

**Box 2.1** The Lamaze care practices to optimise normal birth

- Let labour begin on its own.
- Walk, move around and change positions throughout labour.
- Bring a loved one, friend or doula for continuous support.
- Avoid interventions that are not medically necessary.
- Avoid giving birth on your back, and follow your body's urges to push.
- Keep mother and baby together – it's best for mother, baby and breastfeeding.

(Lothian and DeVries 2005)

---

The Bradley Method (Bradley 2008) has championed the role of fathers in supporting their partner through labour and birth. Fundamentally, he is to be a coach, supporter and encourager for his partner in enabling her to have a natural birth with minimal intervention. Robert Bradley, a physician in the USA, developed this approach as a counter to the use of general anaesthetics and 'twilight sleep' that was widespread in the 1960s. He championed the presence of male partners at the labour and birth but only on the condition that they undertook instruction on how to support their partner through a drug-free labour. His approach was to foreshadow the extensive body of research from the 1970s onwards on the key role of doulas in birth, though those studied were exclusively female companions. In fact, theories evolved in the 1990s suggesting women were much more those studied were exclusively female companions. In fact, theories evolved in the 1990s suggesting women were much more effective in this role because of their 'tend and befriend' instead of 'fight or flight' response to stress (Taylor *et al.* 2000). It was not until 2010 that evidence began to emerge that was supportive of the father's presence at birth (Kainz *et al.* 2010). The Bradley Method subsequently broadened out to include training for all birth companions. The method is built around the six needs of labouring women: darkness and solitude, physical comfort during the first stage of labour, physical relaxation, controlled breathing, need for closed eyes and the appearance of sleep (Bradley 2008).

The Active Birth Movement was initiated by Janet Balaskas in the late 1970s and went on to be hugely influential in the UK in particular. She published the Active Birth Manifesto in 1982 and has been campaigning for the natural childbirth cause since that time. Her book, *New Active Birth* (1990), was read by many midwives, and she spoke with clarity and conviction about the need for upright birth positions, using the evocative metaphor of the 'stranded beetle position' to illustrate much of what was going on in hospital birth. An active birth philosophy has increasingly been adopted by antenatal education curricula, especially in birth centres and midwifery-led units. Though the focus is principally on movement and posture for birth, the underlying philosophy encourages women to take charge of their labour by developing birth plans, thereby exercising autonomy in decision-making.

The National Childbirth Trust began in the late 1950s as an interest group to explore natural childbirth as advocated by Dick-Read and has grown into the largest UK charity addressing parenting and childbirth issues. Now known as the NCT, it has a national network of educators and instructors running parent and antenatal education across the country (NCT 2010). It has long had a campaigning agenda, challenging labour and birth interventions over the past forty years. From confronting routine policies on episiotomy and artificial rupture of membranes in labour (Kitzinger 1990) to recent initiatives to improve home birth provision and the birth environments of hospitals (Newburn and Singh 2004), the NCT has been at the forefront of UK maternity service reform.

Although it has been criticised for attracting a particular demographic to its classes, in recent years the NCT has been providing NHS antenatal education packages, widening its constituency. Educationally, it has adopted adult education principles with small groups, a client-led agenda and a belief in building up long-term networks. During the 1970s and 1980s, like many NHS classes it endorsed and taught psychoprophylaxis, borrowing from Lamaze, but it has evolved into a range of provision today, including yoga and hypno-birthing.

## Focus of educational content and evidence base

Antenatal education across the Western world has always attempted to marry a focus on labour and birth with a focus on early parenting skills, albeit the latter generally limited to baby feeding issues and baby care. To some extent this has been an uneasy pairing because many teachers say that labour concerns dominate clients' interests up to the birth and getting them to focus on life with a baby before that event is difficult. Curricular content is delivered typically over a 6–8-week period, straddling the last trimester for most women. NHS provision in the UK has traditionally been professional-led, both in content and delivery. Although it has always been seen as a core attribute of the midwife's role, many midwives would say it is an aspect of the job they don't particularly enjoy, while a minority embrace it fully. Arguably, speaking to and facilitating groups is an acquired skill that some midwives have more of an aptitude for than others.

Though provision has been traditionally widespread across the UK, it is known that most attendees are women experiencing their first baby, and, of that cohort, less than 50 per cent actually book on to courses (Nolan 2005). The service therefore has been criticised as being elitist and self-selecting. However, it is probably the absence of good-quality evidence that attending classes makes any difference to an individual's labour and birth experience that creates ambivalence for maternity service managers. A number of reviews of studies have shown this lack of effect, including Gagnon and Sandall's (2007) Cochrane review. They conclude: 'the effects of general antenatal education for childbirth or parenthood, or both, remain largely unknown.' Nolan (2005) came to the same conclusion in her doctoral work in this area. The Department of Health commissioned a review more recently, the results of which were published by McMillan *et al.* in 2009, entitled *Birth and Beyond*. In the most comprehensive review of available evidence to date – including examining specialist subgroups with risk factors, preparation for parenthood as a specific subsection, preparation for infant feeding, prevention of depression and preparation for fathers – they concurred with other reviewers. On labour and birth they state that there is little evidence that traditional childbirth classes reduce pain or epidurals or increase the incidence of normal birth. However, attendance is associated with higher levels of satisfaction with the birth experience.

Much of the literature on education packages is confounded by the heterogeneity of the packages of care: differing objectives (labour, parenting, building networks); differing providers (lay and professional); differing methods (curriculum content, size of classes, numbers of classes); differing target audience (low risk, high risk, teenagers, fathers included).

Since 2009, there have been two studies that have focused just on reducing birth interventions, with contrasting results. Interestingly, they were both published in an obstetric, rather than a midwifery, journal. Bergström and colleagues (2009) tested a natural childbirth education package against standard antenatal education in various Swedish maternity hospitals via a randomised controlled trial (RCT). They found no difference in epidural rates between the two. Maimburg *et al.* (2010) subjected a 'Ready for Child' antenatal education package to an RCT, comparing with no antenatal education, and found that the recipients of 'Ready for Child' presented later in labour and had fewer epidurals than the latter group, though no less pain relief overall. Foster (2005) conducted an audit of a 'Birthtalk' package of antenatal education in a large UK maternity unit which halved the epidural rate and doubled the upright posture rate in a group of nulliparous women. The characteristics of the package were:

- small numbers of couples (five or six);
- took place in a typical birth room that women would use for labour;
- participant-led;
- held at around 34–36 weeks' gestation;
- facilitated by labour ward midwives who would be caring for the women when they arrived in labour.

Foster (2005) speculates that it was the combination of these factors that resulted in the favourable outcomes. Certainly, it was able to address a criticism of many antenatal classes that there is a gap between what is taught and what it experienced.

In summary, there is tentative evidence that specific antenatal education packages may make a difference to labour and birth interventions. Over the past five years, quite specific therapies and new approaches to antenatal care provision are beginning to demonstrate more dramatic differences, and I will turn to these next.

## Specific therapies and new approaches to antenatal care provision

Walker *et al.* (2009) discussed some of these newer approaches based in singular techniques and therapies, including hypno-birthing and mindfulness. Hypno-birthing originated in the USA with Marie Mongan (2005), who focused on the use of language as the primary mechanism to reduce anxiety and build confidence in the birth process. For example, the words 'contractions' and 'pain' are replaced by 'surges'. There is a focus on

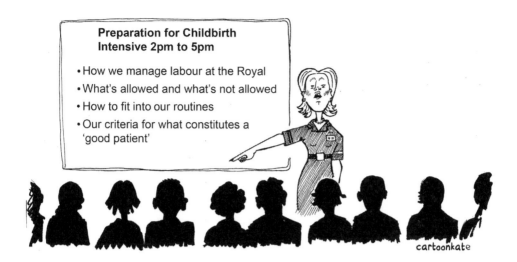

achieving deep relaxation through breathing and visualisation. Birth companions are encouraged to take on coaching roles in supporting their partners. Though this approach has not been researched as an antenatal package, other forms of hypnosis applied in labour do have a substantial evidence base (Smith *et al.* 2006, Cyna *et al.* 2004), demonstrating a reduction in epidurals and narcotics and greater satisfaction with pain management. In addition, there are many anecdotes from midwives that self-hypnosis is very helpful for the latent phase of labour, reducing early labour admissions.

Closely related to hypno-birthing is neuro-linguistic programming (NLP), which again is beginning to accumulate anecdotes about its usefulness for labour. Camm (2006) wrote about its use by individual midwives who were very positive about its ability as a technique to support women in labour. Harnessing the power of language and visualisation, it works by reframing negative anticipated or past experience as positive.

Another approach from this stable of therapies is Mindfulness-Based Stress Reduction, which 'cultivates moment-to-moment non-judgemental awareness of one's present experience through meditation' (Walker *et al.* 2009, p. 473). Already proven as evidence-based in reducing anxiety (Speca *et al.* 2000), mindfulness's application to labour deals with the problem of anticipatory anxiety, encouraging the childbearing woman to 'live in the present moment'.

The therapeutic benefits of water immersion in reducing epidural use are well established (Cluett and Burns 2009, Da Silva *et al.* 2009), with the additional benefit of facilitating labour progress (Zanetti-Dällenbach *et al.* 2006). Though there is no research on aquanatal antenatal classes, the first book on this topic has been published recently (Baines and Murphy 2010). Those running aquanatal antenatal classes testify to the fact that many of these women choose water immersion for labour and therefore presumably benefit from these effects. I would tentatively suggest that aquanatal classes should be placed within the broad category of preparation for childbirth education.

Finally, in relation to specific therapies, the first RCT of a yoga exercise regime during pregnancy revealed an association with shorter labour and less pain, though this did not reduce augmentation and analgesia use in labour (Chuntharapat *et al.* 2008).

The idea of including preparation for childbirth education within the context of normal antenatal care and contacts has been taken up by the CenteringPregnancy programme (Teate *et al.* 2009). Women meet in groups of around ten, facilitated by a midwife with an emphasis on education around pregnancy, birth and parenting, though this is very participant-led. This innovative approach has an impressive evidence base arising from a major RCT in the USA. Ickovics *et al.* (2007) found a lowering of preterm birth rates, significantly better prenatal knowledge, with women feeling more ready for labour and delivery and having greater satisfaction with care, and higher breastfeeding initiation rates. Because the programme emphasises group interaction and solidarity, it builds social capital and communities of women who tend to stay in contact beyond the birth (Wedin *et al.* 2008). To read in greater depth differences between CenteringPregnancy group antenatal classes and traditional childbirth education classes, I would recommend Walker and Worrell (2008).

Within caseload midwifery schemes, the thirty-six-week birth talk at home is another alternative approach that builds on the relationship context of caseload care and continuity through the intrapartum phase. This visit can last up to an hour-and-a-half, with a thorough discussion about all aspects of labour and birth. Kemp and Sandall (2008) coined the phrase 'magical birth' to capture what women said about the 36-week birth talk which was clearly predicated on a desire to maximise normality. This approach echoes what most of these models premise their educational strategy on – a desire to work with normal birth physiology to optimise its expression within a culture that tends to medicalise it.

## New directions and conclusion

The content of this chapter has largely focused on education for birth itself, though preparation for parenthood has been alluded to throughout. It appears this is more challenging to address antenatally, but a recent policy emphasis on parenting, including specifically fathering, has challenged providers to address these areas. With the advent of the Fatherhood Institute and the publication of its *The Dad Deficit: The Missing Piece in the Maternity Jigsaw* (2009), there is now a charity working to raise awareness, provide training and encourage research into the contribution fathers can make through all phases of care. Deave and colleagues (2008) have revealed the pressures on relationships that new parenting brings and urge education and preparation for this area. Recent research into fathers' postnatal depression (up to 10 per cent incidence) and its negative effects on maternal depression (Paulson and Bazemore 2010) further emphasise the importance of addressing these needs. Perhaps the most promising programme for addressing preparation for parenting is PIPPIN (Parr 1997). The programme led to an increase in psychological well-being, parental confidence, satisfaction with the partner relationship and satisfaction with the parent–infant relationship in the postnatal period.

For maternity services faced with increasing pressure for routine interventions like epidurals and induction of labour, some of which is coming from women themselves, antenatal education takes on a crucial role in presenting and equipping women and their partners for an alternative. Such education provides the opportunity for a discussion of a philosophy towards birth that values physiology and is fully aware of the complication of birth interventions. It also needs to include the opportunity to explore and train in a range of other therapeutic approaches that are known to reduce reliance on pain-relieving drugs. Many of these have been outlined above and most do not require extensive training for the midwife. They are relatively low in cost, yet have the potential to make a major impact on labour interventions.

It is therefore disappointing to see the maternity services, at least in the UK, under-investing in antenatal education. Though this has provided a niche for many private providers, their services are fee-paying and potentially exclude the groups that may benefit the most. It is short-sighted to cut investment in this area when emerging evidence is beginning to show real benefit to women. What is needed urgently is reprioritising of education antenatally that focuses on providing a range of these therapeutic options. The mode of their delivery can be variable as long as they adopt adult education best-practice principles. No longer can service providers lament undesirable trends in intrapartum care if they are not prepared to invest in preventive strategies during the antenatal period. Preparation for childbirth and parenting has enormous potential to change the face of intrapartum care for the better. It is an opportunity that should not be spurned.

## Practice recommendations

- Maternity services should have established services for delivering preparation for childbirth and parenting educational packages.
- Such packages should be based on adult education principles of participatory, learner-led models.
- Packages should address the current gap between what is taught and what is experienced.
- Packages should include or inform participants of the range of psychological, sensory, physical and complementary therapies that can aid preparation.
- Primary care midwives have an ongoing responsibility to address education needs during the antenatal period.

### Questions for reflection

What is the current provision of antenatal education like where you work?

How many of the therapeutic approaches mentioned in this chapter are available in your local area?

Can you think of ways that the content and method of delivery could be improved?

How could better training in therapeutic approaches be provided for midwives?

# Chapter 3    **Birth setting and environment**

- Out-of-hospital birth: home birth
- Out-of-hospital birth: free-standing birth centres
- Integrated birth centres/MLUs
- Attitudes and beliefs
- Relational dimensions of care
- Birth ecology, birth territory and midwifery guardianship
- Conclusion
- Practice recommendations
- Questions for reflection

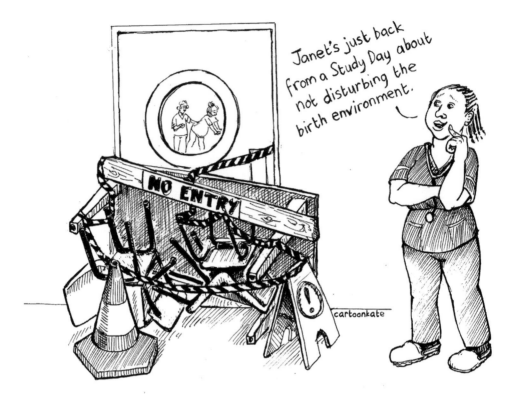

In this chapter I want to examine and discuss the place of birth (home, free-standing birth centres, integrated birth centres/midwifery-led units, obstetric-led labour wards), style of birth (beliefs/attitudes of women and staff, relational models of care), the choice of birth companions and finally some thoughts on the immediate physical surrounds or birth ecology.

The setting for birth is immensely powerful and can be the difference between a fulfilling and a traumatic childbirth experience. Kirkham (2005) engaged with this truism when she challenged midwives at an International Conference of Midwives to think outside the box when confronted by women whose labours slow or stop in hospital. She suggested that transferring women back home when their labour 'malfunctioned' might be the most appropriate action. Her contextual reading of events, probably considered anathema by many hospital-based childbirth professionals, has much to teach us about childbirth and a facilitatory environment.

### Out-of-hospital birth: home birth

The home versus hospital debate shows no signs of abating. Newspapers invariably pick up on journal papers that suggest home birth is unsafe

(Ramesh 2010), most recently Wax and colleagues' (2010) review of planned home birth which concluded that neonatal deaths were tripled by the choice of home, from four births per 1000 in hospital to 15/1000 at home. Critics have pointed to flaws in this paper such as the exclusion of seminal papers for no apparent reason and the inclusion of papers with substandard methods, as well as the use of neonatal mortality rates, rather than the more universally recognised perinatal mortality rates, as the principal outcome measure (Gyte *et al.* 2010). The latter showed no difference between home and hospital. In a similar vein, Symon *et al.*'s (2009) paper got in the headlines when it revealed higher perinatal mortality rates with independent midwives in the UK, even though these were confined to high-risk cases. Both of these studies showed lower labour intervention rates at home. By way of contrast, De Jonge *et al.*'s (2009) nationwide cohort study in the Netherlands of over 500,000 births that showed no difference in perinatal and neonatal mortality between home and hospital never made the headlines, nor did Janssen *et al.*'s (2009) smaller Canadian study revealing a lower perinatal mortality rate at home. It is reasonable to conclude that if the outcomes are good for home birth, they simply don't make it into the newspapers. I have been personally convinced of the safety of home birth since the 1990s, when Tew (1998) and Campbell (1997) conducted their seminal reviews of epidemiological studies which all concluded that home was as safe as hospital for low-risk women. I am therefore less tolerant of the stereotyped response of those who quote the rare catastrophic event argument. However, it is worth restating Tew and Campbell's main argument because it continues to have relevance for other areas of maternity care.

Their most telling argument has always been that concerning public health. Perinatal and maternal mortality did fall dramatically from the 1960s onwards in the UK, but this was because women's health and living conditions improved so dramatically around this time. It was coincidence that the movement of birth into hospital occurred concurrently and to link the two is an error of correlation. I will return to this argument throughout the book because a number of other morbidities (prolonged labour, bleeding during the third stage) take on a different significance when women's intrinsic health status is optimum. Risk factors to take into account when counselling women against home birth continue to multiply with age and obesity becoming prominent in recent years. Throwing light on the increasing pathologisation of labour is a fascinating paper from the Netherlands tracking obstetric referral and involvement in childbirth over a fifty-year period (Amelink-Verburg and Buitendijk 2010). The number of conditions requiring obstetric review and defined in national referral guidelines increased from thirty-nine in 1958 to 143 in 2003, and the odds of an obstetrician being involved in the birth process increased from 24.7 per cent in 1964 to 59.4 per cent in 2002, reflecting this changed referral pattern. It is likely that similar patterns have occurred in other Western countries.

To complete an updating of home birth research published since 2007, studies by Lindgren *et al.* (2008a) and Maassen *et al.* (2008) should be mentioned. Both of these found a statistically significant trend to lower caesarean and assisted vaginal birth rates in home birth groups, with the former demonstrating a lower incidence of anal sphincter tears at home. Olsen and Jewell's (2009) current Cochrane review concludes:

> the change to planned hospital birth for low risk pregnant women in many countries during this century was not supported by good evidence. Planned hospital birth may even increase unnecessary interventions and complications without any benefit for low risk women. With the data currently available one could argue that for low risk pregnancies both home and hospital births *are sufficiently safe for safety no longer to be of overriding importance.*
>
> (my emphasis)

There are many childbirth professionals and childbirth activists who would welcome a release from the constant spurious arguments around home birth and safety and the possibility of shifting the focus to the *lived experience of home birth*. This is the territory that advocates for years have been stressing holds the key to the real home birth dividend: to do with empowerment, healing, egalitarian relationships with carers, opportunities to express spirituality and sexuality and a reclaiming of the language of emotion around birth (www.homebirth.org.uk): in effect, the fleshing out of a social model of birth, stripped of medicalisation, bureaucratisation and institutionalisation (Kitzinger 2002).

Choosing a home birth within a society where the rate is less than 1 per cent in some places is a political statement. Read Cheyney's (2008) inspiring record of home birth experiences in the USA to fully appreciate this. She concludes, home births

> involve challenging established forms of authoritative knowledge, valuing alternative and more embodied or intuitive ways of knowing, and knowledge sharing through the informed consent process. Adherence to subjugated discourses combined with lived experiences of personal power and the cultivation of intimacy in the birthplace fuel homebirth not only as a minority social movement, but also as a form of systems-challenging praxis.
>
> (p. 2540)

Choosing a home birth critiques the industrial model of large hospital birth and women may do it to achieve the additional evidence-based benefits of continuity of care and carer and having a midwife as the lead professional (Homer *et al.* 2001). These represent additional organisational advantages that should be part of the midwife's information about home birth.

The fact that home birth is such a marginalised choice in current maternity services means that many midwives may never have the opportunity to attend them and this has clear implications for their skills and experience. These are additional reasons why improving the availability of provision is so important. Student midwives and practising midwives need opportunities to see them regularly to address the 'fish can't see water' syndrome of modern maternity services (Wagner 2001). Marsden Wagner's metaphor refers to blindness generated by constant exposure to one way of doing birth so that it becomes normative in the practitioner's experience, rendering her unable to envisage or appreciate any alternative. The Midwives Association of North America (MANA) recognised this pitfall when they developed their pre-registration qualification for midwifery. With their strong roots in apprenticeship-style training, they made it mandatory for students to attend ten out-of-hospital births, at home or at birth centres (www.narm.org/edcategories.htm#meac).

There are relatively straightforward steps services can take to provide more opportunity for women to choose the home birth option:

- offer home birth as an explicit option at booking, with freedom to revisit the possibility during pregnancy;
- leave final decision regarding place of birth until labour.

Alongside these changes, in-house training in home birth skills should be mandatory for all clinical midwives. It is as least as important as the current mandatory requirement for emergency skill drills and more important than training in CTG interpretation.

## Out-of-hospital birth: free-standing birth centres

Birth centres and midwifery-led units (MLUs) have become a central agenda item in maternity services in recent years. This is because the continued merger of small maternity hospitals, forming mega-hospitals of 6000+ births per year, has opened up the possibility of siting birth centres where previously the small hospitals stood. Another reason for their profile is the media coverage of closure threats in a variety of localities in the UK, USA and Australia. In fact the growth of lobby groups, clustered around the common cause of birth centres, is a phenomenon in itself with alliances of midwives, users and local politicians displaying impressive and successful politically sophisticated strategies (Walsh 2005).

This interest in birth centres has generated research with a number of papers being published in recent years, both quantitative (Laws *et al.* 2010) and qualitative (Walsh 2007, Thorgen and Crang-Svalenius 2009).

Though the quantitative papers have been criticised for their rigour (Stewart *et al.* 2004), studies conclude that the direction of findings favour birth centres regarding birth interventions (Walsh and Downe 2004, Reddy *et al.* 2004). Jackson *et al.* (2003b) additionally concluded that these facilities were also cheaper to run. Reassurance on safety comes from a recent Australian study examining outcomes of women who intended to birth in birth centres compared with low-risk women choosing maternity hospitals. Both have very low perinatal mortality rates but the latter group had more birth interventions, higher rates of admission to neonatal units and of preterm birth and low birth weight (Laws *et al.* 2010).

Studies of free-standing birth centres (FSBCs) are confounded by selection bias of their potential clients (mostly middle class and well educated). However, a fascinating US study reviewed outcomes from a birth centre that women had not chosen but were forced to attend because the host hospital was full (Scupholme and Kamons 1987). Lower intervention rates persisted during this time, suggesting other factors are operating here as well as maternal preference. Hints of what this could be are offered in an ethnographic study of a New York birth centre (Esposito 1999). Women in this study were disillusioned with childbirth after their first hospital experience but over the course of their pregnancies internalised the active birth philosophy of the birth centre staff and went on to have empowering birth experiences in the main. Green and colleagues (1998), in elucidating this point, uncovered the key role of expectations in shaping birth experiences in their large survey of UK women, concluding that those who entered the labour event with optimism did better than those with prior negative presuppositions. Apparently, midwives at the New York birth centre were able, via antenatal contact with women, to gently challenge the women's prior negative expectations and assist them in adopting a more positive outlook. This is a very exciting finding for midwives burdened by women's pessimism and fear about childbirth events, as it suggests there is a window of opportunity antenatally to work with these attitudes.

My own ethnography of an English FSBC revealed organisational, architectural and attitudinal features of these environments that help promote physiological birth (Walsh 2006a and b). The organisational features mostly relate to scale and temporal effects. Neither women nor midwives felt pressured to be processed or to process women through the birth centre, allowing time for the unfolding of labour events. This released the staff from a 'doing to' ethic, and enabled a 'being with' disposition to express itself. This freedom occurred because, with about 300 births per year, it was rare for there to be more than one woman in labour at any one time. As a midwife familiar with the assembly-line of large hospital birth, this was a refreshing and insightful experience. I saw midwives practising humane, compassionate midwifery and witnessed some wonderful physiological, non-interventionist births, especially of primigravid women.

The staff at the birth centre had a central focus on honing the birth environment to maximise the potential for normal birth. They were constantly making over the birth room decor. Women really appreciated this ambience, which appeared central to their decisions to choose to give birth there. I believe I was seeing the overt expression of a 'nesting instinct' that, though clearly manifest in mammals, is latent in humans because medically managed birth has suppressed it (Johnston 2004). When given the freedom to surface, it expressed itself in a complex weave of environmental and emotional ambience reading. At the same time, women reconceptualised safety as having a psychosocial dimension in a move away from the traditional morbidity/mortality focus. Both architectural and attitudinal components contributed to this new way of seeing (Walsh 2006a).

Traditional understandings of evidence do not accommodate these differing influences on clinical practice and the experience of care, and are therefore unable to detect the subtle nuances affecting a complex phenomenon like childbirth.

Finally, other interesting dimensions of birth centre care are to do with their interface with secondary and tertiary services. There is the question of intrapartum transfers, regarding both the rates of transfer and the process of transfer. Rates vary enormously from 3 per cent to 25 per cent in some studies (Reddy et al. 2004). There are multiple factors at work here, among them the original booking criteria and the experience of birth centre midwives. Rowe's (2010) recent appraisal of various maternity services' criteria for transfer revealed a distinct lack of robustness in their development and application and this is an area that clearly needs to be addressed with some urgency.

Research into the process of transfer has already alerted us to the sometimes dysfunctional interface at handover between birth centre and host unit. Annandale's (1988) study showed the liability of having a host unit that is hostile and whose overt message is: 'the only time we see you is when we are sorting out your disasters.' In an interesting analogy with home birth intrapartum transfer, Davis-Floyd (2003) wrote of 'disarticulation' at this interface where the home birth midwife's story is discounted and discredited by hospital staff who rate their own knowledge as authoritative. Within the UK, the forthcoming *Birthplace* study (NPEU 2011), which is examining these factors in some depth, is eagerly anticipated. As well as tracking referral patterns for the first time systematically, qualitative research is examining women's experience. There are enough incidences of closer scrutiny when a bad outcome occurs in an FSBC than when one occurs in a large hospital to argue for major efforts to be made in promoting positive relationships and greater understanding between the two. I will make some suggestions for these after the next section on integrated birth centres.

FSBCs are the closest ideologically to home birth than all other models for low-risk labour care. Along with home birth, there are many reasons why they could be the 'default option' for the majority of normal births. However, like home birth they are a soft option for marginalisation and the deprioritising in provision driven by economic rationalism which perceives that the centralisation of birth delivers economies-of-scale benefits. This perception persists despite good evidence that size becomes self-defeating once bed provision exceeds certain levels (Posnett 1999). The other principal driver in Western maternity services is the regionalisation of neonatal services so that intensive care facilities are concentrated in tertiary referral centres. In the UK, this has led to the closure of small neonatal facilities and smaller maternity units (Shribman 2007). In some metropolitan areas, this has led to the opening of FSBCs to provide local birthing facilities for local women. Despite this, the profile of FSBCs tends to be low, except in their local communities where they tend to provide their services largely unheard and unseen until they are threatened with closure. Then frequently they fight courageous, protracted campaigns on a 'small is beautiful' ticket with mixed results. Readers are encouraged to read Deery *et al.*'s (2010) recent book on such a struggle.

## Integrated birth centres/MLUs

It's difficult to understand why integrated birth centres have not become commonplace as birth has become more centralised. As a model, they have had a substantial orthodox evidence base with their own Cochrane systematic review since the late 1990s. During the 1980s and 1990s, randomised trials (RCTs) were undertaken in a number of Western countries (Sweden, Australia, UK, Ireland and Canada) on this model, showing more normal birth, better breastfeeding initiation, a reduction in epidural, oxytocin augmentation and episiotomy rates, higher levels of maternal satisfaction and no statistical difference in perinatal mortality (Hodnett *et al.* 2010). In fact, Hodnett's updated Cochrane review changed its conclusion away from earlier concerns about a trend to higher perinatal mortality in birth centres. Now the meta-analysis, incorporating some new studies, shows no difference in that outcome between birth centres and hospitals regarding perinatal mortality.

All of these settings established their birth centres with geographical separation from the main labour ward: partitioned on the same wing, a different wing, a different floor or occasionally a different building. This is understood to be fundamental to the success of the model as it allows for the evolution of distinct philosophies and the possibility of different staffing, which promotes ownership and consistency in care. Ethnographic studies of large obstetric-led labour wards have revealed their hierarchical, institutional and medically led ethos (Hunt and Symonds 1995, Machin and Scamell 1997, Thorgen and Crang-Svalenius 2009) that make the carving out of a 'birth as normal' space in their midst problematic indeed. From time to time, both midwifery and obstetric voices suggest that separate spaces will destroy teamwork and collaboration but this has always struck me as a fundamental misunderstanding of what multi-disciplinary working means. It does not mean doing everything together, but working independently to each other's strengths and collaborating where interface naturally occurs. Not being in each other's pockets does not negate the possibility of constructive cooperation when needed. Second, euphemisms about teamwork have too often in the past masked unhelpful power differentials between midwives and obstetricians that left midwives feeling oppressed, as Kirkham's team of researchers have constantly reminded us (Kirkham 1999, Ball *et al.* 2002, Stapleton *et al.* 2002).

One criticism of separating birth centres from traditional labour wards is that the former tend to receive all the investment in environmental upgrade. A much better approach is to upgrade the decor and facilities of labour wards in line with similar changes in birth centres, especially in the provision of birthing pools which are being increasingly used for their water immersion benefits in higher-risk women.

Additional suggestions to improve the interface between birth centres and host labour wards are: to have regular reviews of transfers, regular reviews of 'best cases' where transfers were averted, regular dissemination of physiological birth markers of good practice and having a link with one obstetrician who is supportive of the model. Leadership in both settings needs to be collaborative and trusting, which sets a template for all other staff.

## Attitudes and beliefs

It seems reasonable to assume that midwives choosing to work in home birth and birth centre settings would be a self-selecting group and that they would exhibit beliefs and practices that are congruent with these environments. However, qualitative research has painted a more complicated picture. Edwards (2000) discovered that some women in her Scottish home birth study experienced a 'hospital birth at home', and Annandale (1987) coined the phrase 'ironic intervention' to represent the action of midwives routinely rupturing membranes in mid-labour to avoid transfer out of a birth centre to a consultant unit for prolonged labour. Machin and Scamell (1997) described the 'irresistible nature of the biomedical metaphor' in explaining how women oriented to normal birth bought into medical interventions once they entered the hospital. It is becoming clear that assumptions cannot be made about the attitudes of midwives or women who choose birth centre options.

Coyle *et al.*'s (2001a and b) papers remind us that women who opt for birth centres expect to be cared for by midwives who share their values around birth. Downe and McCourt (2008) espouse the importance of a focus on positive outcomes of birth, rather than on morbidity, captured in the term 'salutogenesis', or well-being. Such a focus is an imperative for birth centre staff, as is a fundamental trust in the physiological processes of labour. This is where an explicit promotion of a philosophy of active birth and of the values behind a social model of care is so important for birth centre work. These approaches explicitly affirm birth physiology and their impact on women antenatally has been demonstrated by Foster's (2005) audit of an antenatal education package based on these beliefs. Women who went through this programme had half the epidural rate of women who did not, confirming for the first time that preparation for childbirth classes can impact on the labour experience.

Because of the current dominance of risk in maternity policy and care (Tracey *et al.* 2007, Dahlen 2010), it is especially appropriate to explore attitudes to risk and normal, physiological birth when appointing staff to birth centre settings. There is mounting evidence that midwives view risks associated with birth along a continuum from normal to high (Regan and Liaschenko 2007) and that the same midwives are more risk-averse with the same women depending on the setting (Crabtree 2008). Dahlen (2010) cogently argues that a heightened awareness of risk increases our sense of fear and the effect of this on childbirth is a predisposition to dystocia and emergency caesarean section (Laursen *et al.* 2009).

Another area where a midwife's attitude may make a significant difference in birth centre care is around the pain of labour. Leap and Anderson (2008) argue convincingly for a 'working with pain' approach to replace the 'pain relief' orientation of most birthing services. As they counsel, the midwife needs to be comfortable with the expression of pain in physiological labours. I will return to this theme in a later chapter.

It is therefore good practice to explore the motivation of midwives who apply for birth centre posts to gain insights into their beliefs and values. But prior to this, the philosophy and strategic direction of the birth centre needs articulating in information leaflets for women and in policy documents. Operationally, the opportunity should be provided antenatally for midwives to meet women who will access the centre for birth, ideally through repeat antenatal clinics or through childbirth education classes.

Facilitating midwifery contact with women antenatally introduces the subject of relational components to care and there is a wealth of research confirming its significance for normal labour and birth.

## Relational dimensions of care

Critiques of the evidence paradigm include its undervaluing of common sense as every aspect of practice is subjected to research scrutiny, even those aspects that just seem appropriate because thoughtful reflection and common sense tells us so (Wickham 1999). This argument could be applied to the research that has examined relational components of midwifery care. Teams, caseloads and continuity of care all, at some level, enshrine the benefit of women establishing a relationship with their carers rather than being cared for by strangers within a fragmented model. It isn't exactly 'rocket science' to intuit that journeying through such a significant rite-of-passage experience as childbirth is best done in the company of known carers. How many times do we have to repeat studies that keep shouting at us that these characteristics of a service are highly valued by women and consistently reduce birth interventions? It was therefore refreshing and challenging to hear a story coming out of South America that a country there has recognised that continuous support in labour is a fundamental human right. They may legislate to make it illegal for maternity services not to provide this dimension to care. After all, they argued, the benefits have been proven again and again, across different countries and different decades.

Nine RCTs in Hodnett *et al.*'s (2011) systematic review concluded that continuous support during labour reduced caesarean sections, pharmacological analgesia, assisted vaginal birth, low Apgar scores and labour length, while women experienced more positive births. In addition, the authors make two telling points:

1 that the most effective support may come from those not employed by the institution;

2 that continuous support will be less effective in a highly medicalised environment.

Rosen (2004) reviewed eight studies of labour support provided by five different categories of person and concluded that care by known, untrained lay-women, starting in early labour, was the most effective. Taylor and colleagues (2000) explained this phenomenon by analysing stress responses in females. In a dramatic echo of childbirth physiology, they found that oxytocin was released in women exposed to stress and this triggered 'tending and befriending' behaviours rather than the classic (male) response of 'fight or flight'. In a further mirroring of the hormonal cascade of labour, endogenous opiates (beta endorphins), also released during the experience of stress, augment these effects.

One could tease out some interesting implications from these findings, including a questioning of the common expectation that the male partner should be the principal birth companion. Midwives have long questioned the wisdom of this practice for some labours where a frightened, non-engaged male presence has had a negative impact. Equally challenging is the finding that non-medically trained people who are external to the institution are more effective at labour support. Research suggests that these individuals are more likely to have built a rapport prior to admission to hospital, are committed to staying with the woman throughout the labour (i.e. cannot be called away to help elsewhere on the delivery suite) and are not institutionally programmed to 'the way things are done here'.

Midwives need to explore with women antenatally the selection of their birth companion, taking into account these findings. It challenges all parties to explore the doula option as the most appropriate person to fulfil this remit.

Aside from the consideration of best birth companion, midwives have argued for decades for one-to-one care in labour so that they can genuinely be 'with woman'. It is likely that this organisational aspect alone would increase normal birth rates substantially. In recent years, more evidence has accrued of the significance of limiting the number of continuous carers a woman has in labour. Gagnon and colleagues (2007) demonstrated that, even when controlling for labour confounders, the more carers a woman had during labour, the more likely she was to have a caesarean section. At the other end of the spectrum, Essex and Pickett (2008) found that unaccompanied women were more likely to experience birth interventions, corroborating the findings from doula studies.

Continuity has been the subject of research and debate in midwifery for over twenty years now. One could be forgiven for concluding: is there any more we can learn? A cursory examination of the wider literature in health reveals there is because, of course, continuity has been of interest for many other areas of the health spectrum. Haggerty *et al.* (2005) summarise the literature as follows:

*   informational continuity (patient story available to all relevant agencies);
*   management continuity (consistent, coherent care);
*   relational continuity (known carers).

All three contribute to a better patient experience and, arguably, better care. Midwifery care has focused more on relational continuity, possibly believing that the other two will follow, though this may not be the case. Nevertheless, a case can be made for this focus because of the unique features of the midwife–woman relationship: its biologically determined longevity, its journey through a major rite-of-passage experience and the intimate nature of its focus.

There are many organisational variants of relational continuity in midwifery services: teams, caseloads, group practices, named midwife etc. There has been enough research done around these options to glean some important lessons:

*   Teams should number no more than six because, as numbers increase, 'a known midwife' becomes 'someone met once or twice' to eventually 'someone spoken of by a colleague' and continuity becomes meaningless (Flint 1993).
*   Continuity between phases, especially having a known midwife for labour, is highly valued by women (Walsh 1999) and reduces labour interventions (Page *et al.* 1999, North Staffs 2000).
*   Limiting the number of carers in caseload schemes so that women, when they go into labour, will know their attending midwives. A recent Dutch study showed this reduces interventions (Fontein 2010). Parallel research in Sweden showed that if a midwife was called out to a home birth woman she did not know, the woman was more likely to be transferred to hospital (Lindgren *et al.* 2008b).

In relation to clinical outcomes and satisfaction with care, team and continuity variants generally reduce labour interventions, including epidural, induction of labour, episiotomy and neonatal resuscitation rates, and improve satisfaction.

Some of these benefits are linked to the role of the midwife as the lead carer because a number of other studies in various countries conclude that midwifery-led services are superior to obstetric-led models when caring for a low-risk group (Hatem *et al.* 2008). In addition, Tracy and Tracy (2003) showed that low-tech, midwife-mediated services are cheaper, challenging the notion that closing FSBCs or under-investing in midwives will save money.

## Birth ecology, birth territory and midwifery guardianship

I want to conclude this chapter with some theoretical and practical reflections on the birth environment, drawing on anthropological sources and indigenous wisdom and Fahy *et al.*'s (2008) relatively new theory of birth territory and midwifery guardianship.

One of the effects of the medicalisation of childbirth has been the colonisation of the birth space so that what was once private and sacred is now public and secular. The site of birth is now a neutral space where it was once literally pregnant with symbolism and meaning. Kitzinger's (2000) timeless record of her journey across different cultures and their birthing practices leave an overwhelming impression that the setting of birth was carefully chosen and constructed so that it 'grounded' women to their ancestral land and to their local community. Many women birthed outside among nature and many more in simple dwellings where they could remain in contact with the earth. Furniture was sparse as unencumbered space was considered a premium, and what was available was facilitatory for posture and positional support. The best birth centres attempt to mimic these features: single-storey buildings with access to private gardens, rooms that can be personalised by women with minimal multipurpose furniture, often without beds (Hodnett *et al.* 2009). Hauck *et al.* (2008) have written about the therapeutic value of Snoezelen rooms that provide a multi-sensorial experience aimed at inducing calm. The guarding of the birth space from threats and intruders was a key role for traditional birth attendants in indigenous birth settings, and birth centres generally do well in addressing this.

It is impossible to do justice to Fahy and colleagues' thoughtful and challenging book in one paragraph. Their theory is multi-dimensional (incorporates how space is used, as well as attitudes of carers) and multi-level (social, psychological, spiritual). It is about who has power in the birth space and whether that power is enabling (integrative) or disabling (disintegrative) for women and midwives. If you are only dipping into their book, read Lepori *et al.*'s chapter on birth architecture and the needs of the moving/feeling/dreaming body in birth. There are plenty of practical tips in there for those planning a make-over of their birth facilities, but a wider reading of this text is well worth it if you want an example of how a holistic approach to birthing can actually be fleshed out.

## Conclusion

Careful consideration and attention to detail of the various dimensions to the birth environment establishes optimum conditions for the labour physiology to unfold. This can then become fundamental to optimising physiological birth and reversing decades of medicalisation. Many Western countries, except for perhaps the Netherlands and New Zealand, have inadequate home birth and birth centre provision. For example, less than 10 per cent of women birth in these settings in the UK (Smith and Smith 2005).

Much of what I go on to discuss in the remaining chapters of this book is dependent on the birth setting and its ambience. It serves to remind us that labour and birth cannot be disassembled into stages without losing a coherence and intrinsic connectivity. To extend Kitzinger's metaphor, there can be no 'dance of labour' without skilled players and a suitable stage.

## Practice recommendations

- Free-standing birth centre provision should be expanded.
- Integrated birth centre provision should be expanded.
- The choice of a home birth should be protected and expanded.
- Model of large consultant unit for all birth should be discontinued.
- Women should have an opportunity to see birth space prior to labour.
- Women should be encouraged to personalise birth space.
- Belief in physiological birth should be explicit in birth centre philosophy and in staff approach.
- Team and continuity schemes should be encouraged.
- Birth centre staff should have opportunity to meet women antenatally.
- 'Known midwife for labour schemes' (caseload model) should be encouraged.
- All labouring women should receive continuous support from a trained birth companion.
- All low-risk women should have the option of booking for midwifery-led care.
- Midwives need training in non-institutional birth skills.

**Questions for reflection**

What is your view of the local choices for place of birth where you live/work?

Is midwifery care organised in such a way to harness the known benefits of continuity of care and carer? Could it be?

How facilitatory for normal birth is the birth environment where you work?

How could a midwifery-led model of care be introduced or strengthened where you work?

How could student midwives develop the confidence and skills to work in non-institutional birth environments?

# Chapter 4    Rhythms in the first stage of labour

For midwives who qualified from the 1970s onwards, the linkage of the words 'labour' and 'progress' is axiomatic. In fact, a defining feature of the last fifty years of labour care has been the preoccupation with the pathology of labour length, so much so that it has become an orthodoxy in intrapartum approaches across the world. In the vast majority of hospital birth, progress is assessed by vaginal examination and the procedure has become synonymous with contemporary labour care. This normative mindset is so powerful that few midwives have had the opportunity to observe labours where no vaginal examinations occur. As practitioners of childbirth, we are blinded to some extent by the era we live in. It is difficult for us to appreciate that for millions of years, childbirth was not so obsessed with labour duration. Gaskin (2003) reminds us of that in her uncovering of the word 'pasmo', meaning labour stopped and everybody went home until it started again. She discovered it in a nineteenth-century Portuguese textbook of midwifery.

In this chapter, I will examine the origins of the 'labour progress' mentality and trace the influences of this approach through to the late 1990s when a backlash began to be felt. Alongside the clinical imperative around length of labour, I will argue, sits an organisational imperative that is about getting women through a large hospital system. I will examine the segmenting of labour into phases (latent, active) to show how the biomedical definitions have caused midwives much anguish as they constantly care for women who don't fit the ideal template. I critique the traditional cervicograph (graphic representation of cervical dilatation over time) element of the partogram, almost universally used across the Western world, and examine research into alternative labour curves that challenge the linear notion of progression.

## Friedman's legacy

Emanuel Friedman was the first to graphically record cervical dilatation over time and measure this in a cohort of women. His work in the mid-1950s became seminal in influencing our understanding of average lengths of labour for primigravid and multigravid women and the sigmoid-shaped Friedman curve was incorporated into obstetric and midwifery textbooks for the next fifty years. The curve represented early, middle and later phases of the first stage of labour and was based on two samples of 200 primigravid women in 1954 (Friedman 1954) and 500 primigravid women a year later (Friedman 1955).

In the early 1970s, Philpott and Castle (1972) added the partogram to labour records and amplified the cervicograph to give guidance for what to do if labours were slow. Using just the active phase of the first stage of labour, they drew an alert line at the 1 cm/hour rate, a transfer line at two hours behind the alert line and an action line two hours behind that. The alert line was a signal to the clinician to monitor closely, the transfer line to literally transfer physically to a major hospital and the action line to rupture membranes and administer an oxytocin infusion. Philpott and Castle were working in remote areas of Rhodesia and were concerned about the disastrous consequences of obstructed labours. Studd (1973) measured cohorts of women admitted to UK hospitals at differing stages of cervical dilatation and plotted their dilatation over time.

All three of these cervicograph variations were adapted and added to by O'Driscoll in his protocol of 'active management of labour' (O'Driscoll and Meagher 1986). This interventionist approach had strict criteria for labour diagnosis and aggressive management of slow progress with early recourse to artificial rupture of membranes and intravenous oxytocin if labour did not progress at 1 cm/hour. The active management of labour protocol was responsible for the convention that labours should adhere to the 1 cm/hour template which is much stricter than Philpott's guideline of the early 1970s. Though the active management of labour went out of fashion during the 1990s when it was realised that the only effective component of the package was continuous support during labour (Frigoletto et al. 1995), its championing of syntocinon for the augmentation of labour has left a significant legacy for intrapartum practice today. Some UK studies show that up to 57 per cent of low-risk primigravid women have their labour augmented with exogenous oxytocin (Mead 2008), suggestive of a collapse in the physiological ability of nulliparous women to labour spontaneously.

## Organisational factors

This clinical imperative that long labours resulted in morbidity may not have gained credence without the changes in organisational structures in how maternity care was delivered, in particular the centralising movement of the second half of the twentieth century. With more and more women giving birth in larger and larger hospitals, there was organisational pressure to process women through delivery suites and postnatal wards. Martin (1987) had railed against assembly-line childbirth in the 1980s but it was not until Perkins' (2004) comprehensive and considered critique of USA maternity care policy that the adoption of an essentially business/industrial model by maternity hospitals has been made so explicit. Perkins cited the Henry Ford car-assembly line as the template for the organisation of USA maternity hospital activity.

I elaborated on this critique in a study of childbirth at an FSBC in the UK (Walsh 2006b). Temporal differences were among the most striking between this setting and maternity hospitals. Women's labours were not on a time line and there was no pressure to free up rooms for new occupants. The corollary of hospitals with time restrictions on labour length is that more women can labour and birth within their space. It comes as little surprise to find that the hospitals still practising active management of labour are among the largest in Europe with over 8000 births/year (Murphy-Lawless 1998). Midwives' anecdotes and ethnographies abound with the pressures that exist in big units to 'get through the work' and deal with the labour 'nigglers' (Hunt and Symonds 1995, Thorgen and Crang-Svalenius 2009).

The time pressures that are applied to women's labours in hospital therefore have their origins in both a clinical and an organisational imperative. These pressures can only be addressed by both revising clinical parameters around normal labour length and by simultaneously reducing the workload on very large labour wards. One of the best ways of achieving the latter is by opening up midwifery-led units or birth centres alongside these existing facilities as suggested in the previous chapter on birth environment.

## An emergent critique

The beginnings of a backlash against the clinical imperative was beginning to appear in the late 1990s when Albers (1999) concluded from her research that nulliparous women's labours were longer than Friedman had said. She found that in a low-risk population of women cared for by midwives in nine different centres in the USA, some active phases of labour were twice the length of Friedman's cohort (17.5 hours versus 8.5 hours for nulliparas and 13.8 hours versus seven hours for multiparas) without any consequent morbidity. Cesario's later study (2004) found a similar average length of labour to Friedman but a wider range of normal. Primiparous women remained in the first stage for up to twenty-six hours and multiparous women for twenty-three hours without adverse effects. A more recent randomised controlled trial (RCT) showed that if prescriptive action lines that limit labour length are used with primigravid women, then over 50 per cent will require intervention. The authors thus called for a review of labour length orthodoxies (Lavender et al. 2006).

Obstetric journals were also beginning to question Friedman's curve. Zhang and colleagues (2002) examined the patterns of cervical dilatation in 1329 nulliparous women and found slower dilatation rates in the active phase, especially before 7cm, where the slowest group were all below Friedman's 1cm/hour threshold. They concluded that current diagnostic criteria for protracted or arrested labour may be too stringent, citing important contextual differences in current practice to Friedman's day. Among these are the medical advances for managing longer labours like exogenous oxytocin, epidural anaesthesia and fetal monitoring which were not available in the 1950s. The availability of these drugs and technologies today arguably make the management of dystocia, when it occurs, safer. I would also argue that the increase in general health of the current generation of women compared with fifty years ago makes them less vulnerable to the effects of long labours. In addition Zhang suggests that the mean increase in maternal body mass and fetal weight is probably contributing to slower labours in the present day.

Zhang, Troendle *et al.* (2010) undertook further research more recently on a sample of women from the 1950s in an attempt to examine what they called the 'natural history of the normal first stage of labour'. This interesting retrospective study observed labour in a low-risk cohort prior to the linear progression model of labour care being in place. Zhang and colleagues argued that the widespread acceptance of this paradigm makes it extremely difficult to study the natural trajectory of labour in the present because restrictions on length and time lines are already universally in place. Their findings from this cohort of sixty years ago built on the earlier 2002 study. The acceleratory phase occurred after 5 cm in multiparous women and after 6 cm in many nulliparous women and labour did not decelerate toward full dilatation as Friedman had suggested. On the basis of this, Zhang and colleagues suggest that the active phase of labour in some women, regardless of parity, starts between 5 and 6 cm and that a slowing in labour after this point needs great vigilance than currently afforded. They restated their view that a parabolic curve of labour was much more realistic than linear versions of cervical dilatation (see Figure 4.1).

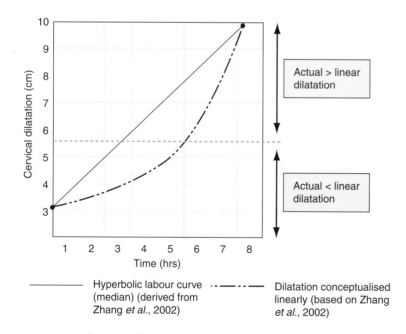

FIGURE 4.1 Zhang *et al.*'s Revised Partogram.

Finally Zhang and colleagues (2010a and b) reviewed data from over 60,000 low-risk parous women between 2005 and 2007 and confirmed all their previous conclusions. Recent observation research by Walsh (2009) also suggest that labours appear to slow on admission prior to 5 cm dilated but not if admission is after 5 cm, indicating that the 5–6 cm mark may be a more accurate reflector of the onset of active labour.

Gurewitsch *et al.*'s (2002) interesting paper contributed newer data on labour rhythms at the other end of parity – grand multiparous women. They found that the latent phase of labour could last till up to 6 cm and that progression after that mimics lower-order parity women, challenging the convention that grand multiparous women labour more quickly.

For an up-to-date summary of all this research, Neal *et al.*'s (2010) paper is excellent. It includes the Zhang hyperbolic labour curve (Figure 4.1) which, if we are to have any graphic to plot labour against, is the best so far.

What all these papers suggest to us is that there is more physiological variation between women than previously thought. Recent criticisms of quantitative research methods (Downe and McCourt 2008) support this. The limitations of methods based on homogenising women statistically towards an average have already been questioned in Chapter 1, but labour progression is a good example. Midwives have always known that many women don't fit the average of a 1 cm/hour dilatation rate and, even more fundamentally, may not physiologically mimic the parameters of the average cervix. Their cervix may be fully dilated at 9 or 11 cm! Given the infinite variety in women's physical appearance and psychosocial characteristics, it seems entirely reasonable to expect subtle differences in their birth physiology.

In recent years a better understanding of the hormones regulating labour has contributed to this more complex picture of physiological variation. Odent (2001) and Buckley (2010) have shown us that the hormonal cocktail influencing these processes is appropriately called the 'dance of labour'. These hormones' delicate interactions mediated by environmental and relational factors resemble the rhythm, beauty and harmony of skilled dancers and I deliberately describe their effects in more metaphorical and poetic language in the following section to counteract the dryness and poverty of the medical language.

Oxytocin is the 'benevolent queen', leading from the front with an array of influences: directly on uterine contractions and in generating feelings of nurture, protection and altruism towards the baby. She orchestrates the dynamic synergy of other hormonal interactions: of the cortisol hormones adrenaline (fight and flight) and noradrenaline (peace-maker), and of the endogenous endorphins. Adrenaline and noradrenaline prepare and empower a woman for the hard labour of birthing by mobilising her strengths and inner resources. With a profound sensitivity, they feed back into oxytocin release to optimise labour progress so that it is neither too fast nor too slow. Their importance is signified by their imbalance: the woman in good labour at home whose stress levels are exacerbated by the journey to hospital stops contracting as excessive adrenaline discharges and becalms oxytocin. This is a reflex action to protect the woman from a potentially hostile environment. Or the woman who, towards the end of long labour, has an epidural. The complete removal of pain stimulates noradrenaline, which wrongly interprets that labour is stopping so feeds back to stop the release of oxytocin so labour is becalmed again.

Then there is the 'inner high' of endogenous endorphins, the hormone of compassion that is secreted when the body is in chronic pain. It also synergises with oxytocin to release it at just the appropriate level to maintain the marriage of the two in progressing the labour while calming the soul.

We are indebted to Odent for highlighting the pivotal role of environment and companions in mediating this magical chemistry of hormonal interaction. These variables can enhance or disturb and the over-diagnosis of 'failure to progress' in hospitals across the world is surely an indictment on a birth setting that is profoundly disturbing for normal labour, especially in a first birth. Odent counsels a reconnecting with the primordial roots of birth, and for this we may need to learn from indigenous cultures where the birth space is sacred space, guarded by birth companions. The hallmarks of this space are privacy and nurturing love above all else. It is no surprise that recent physiology of female companionship under duress reveals a 'tending and befriending' behaviour as opposed to a 'fight or flight' response, and that the kernel for this action is our benevolent queen of hormones, oxytocin (Taylor *et al.* 2000). In a poignant congruence with birth physiology and the labouring woman, it is released in the female birth companions in their work of support. More recent research by Moberg (2004) indicates that oxytocin is secreted in both women and men through therapeutic touch, and, of course, touch is one of the most common expressions of support by birth companions.

## Rhythms in early labour

The division of the first stage of labour into latent and active is clinician-based and not necessarily resonant with the lived experience of labour, as women with long latent phases have been trying to tell us for ages. The progress template has led us down a distinctly non-woman-centred cul-de-sac here. We cannot, when she comes into hospital, validate her description of labour pains for seven days because we dare not record a length of labour greater than twenty-four hours. We therefore invent euphemisms for her experience that allows us to classify her story as not being genuine labour – spurious labour, false labour or, simply and starkly, 'you're not in labour'. The negative consequences this has for women's morale and confidence are now well established (Eri *et al.* 2009, Barnett *et al.* 2008, Carlsson *et al.* 2009). Gross and colleagues (2003, 2006) have illuminated our understanding of the phenomenon of early labour by revealing how eclectically it presents in different women and how women vary in their self-diagnosis. Less than 60 per cent of women experienced contractions as the starting point of their labours. The remainder described fluid loss (28 per cent), constant pain (24 per cent), blood-stained loss (16 per cent), gastrointestinal symptoms (6 per cent), emotional upheaval (6 per cent) and sleep alterations (4 per cent) as heralding the start of labour, none of which fits the classic textbook definition. Gross suggests we change the direction of our questioning from eliciting the pattern of contractions to simply enquiring 'how did you recognise the start of labour'?

Eri *et al.* (2009) and Cheyne *et al.* (2006) point out that the midwifery diagnosis of labour in hospital is not simply a unilateral clinical judgement but a complex blend of balancing the totality of the woman's situation with institutional constraints like workloads, guidelines, continuity concerns, justifying decisions to senior staff and risk management. Contrast this with care at a home birth or FSBC where the organisational and clinical parameters are secondary to women's lived experience and care is driven by the latter (Walsh 2006a).

Twenty years ago, Flint (1986) counselled that early labour was best experienced at home with access to a midwife, and a recent trial confirms that this remains the ideal (Janssen *et al.* 2003). Maternity services now know that the worst place to be is on a labour ward because, as recent research shows, women just end up having more labour interventions (Bailit *et al.* 2005, Rahnama *et al.* 2006). This is because of the organisational imperative of processing women through the system. Recent studies have shown the value of triage facilities or early labour assessment centres if home assessment in early labour is not an option. Women who attend them have fewer labour interventions (Lauzon and Hodnett 2001). Jackson *et al.* (2003b) counselled the value of attending an FSBC and Turnbull *et al.* (1996) of seeing a midwife and not an obstetrician. Individualising care and ongoing informational and relational continuity are all important elements of best practice for the latent phase of labour. For an excellent and fuller discussion of latent phase of labour, see McDonald's (2010) paper in the *British Journal of Midwifery*.

## Rhythms in mid-labour

As I have already mentioned, Philpott and Castle invented the partogram in the early 1970s and it has become a ubiquitous aspect of labour care ever since, endorsed by national guideline groups (NICE 2007) and the World Health Organisation (WHO 1994). Therefore I was amazed to discover that Lavender *et al.*'s (2008) systematic review concluded 'we cannot recommend routine use of the partogram as part of standard labour management and care' (p. 2). Five RCTs involving 6000 women showed no difference in caesarean section rates and other morbidities between partogram and no partogram. I have only come across two clinical settings where partograms were not a routine element of care and those were home birth and FSBC settings. If this graphic portrayal of labour had not been adopted across the Western world, it is possible that the labour progress paradigm would not have become so entrenched.

I have discussed the relaxation in time lines around this issue and now want to explore the decoupling of the phenomenon of labour slowing or stopping from the presumption that it always represents pathology. Apart from strong anecdotal evidence that some women experience a latent period in the middle of their labour, it was not until Davis *et al.*'s (2002) paper on labour 'plateaus' that statistical data was available (Figure 4.2).

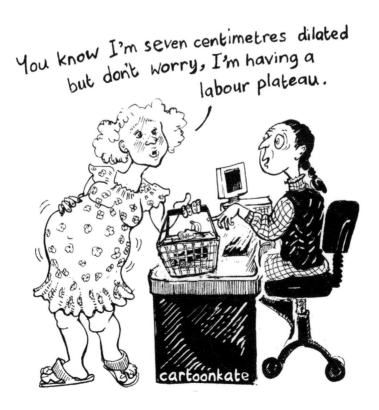

47

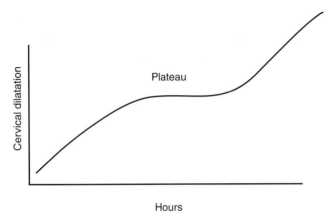

Cervical dilatation

Plateau

Hours

FIGURE 4.2 The MANA Curve.

Their retrospective examination of thousands of records of home birth women discovered that some had periods when the cervix stopped dilating temporarily in active labour in response to a quiescent period in uterine activity. This was not interpreted as pathology by their birth attendants, and after variable periods of time, cervical progression began again as contractions came back. A similar scenario has been described in birth centres (Walsh 2006c) where women appear to 'stop' their labours to deal with concerns that they have, for example completing a task that needed doing before the baby arrives, waiting for birth companions to arrive. Gaskin's description of 'pasmo' indicated that physiological delays were known about in the nineteenth century. An important differentiating element is that cervical dilatation stops as contractions go off. I am not suggesting that if contractions are intense, frequent and regular that cessation in cervical dilatation can be ignored: that situation may indicate an underlying problem like posterior position or a true dystocia.

With this new understanding of the subtlety of hormonal interactions and the mediating effects of environment and companions, we can then engage with the individuality of the labour experience for different women. It then becomes entirely feasible that actually labour could be understood as a 'unique normality', varying from woman to woman (Downe and McCourt 2008). Midwifery skill lies in facilitating its individual expression in women in our care.

Recent research into the use of differing action lines (two hours and four hours behind the 1 cm/hour line) in the active phase of labour has shown that allowing for a slower rate of cervical dilatation (four hours behind the 1 cm/hour alert line) does not result in more caesarean sections and, importantly, women were just as satisfied with longer labours (Lavender *et al.*

2006). The *Guide to Effective Care in Pregnancy and Childbirth* (Enkin *et al*. 2000) now recommends a cervical dilatation rate of 0.5 cm/hour in nulliparous women and this has been endorsed by the NICE intrapartum guideline (NICE 2007).

The ubiquity of vaginal examination as a practice in labour is inextricably linked to the progress paradigm. It deserves some appraisal as a common childbirth intervention to see if its widespread use is justifiable. It clearly does not pass Enkin *et al*.'s (2000) first test that any labour intervention should either enhance normal physiological processes or correct a deviation from the normal. Devane's (1996) systematic literature review fails to identify the research basis for this procedure, which reveals the power of the labour progress paradigm, effectively driving the adoption of the procedure on the basis of custom and practice. It also fails the second test of minimal untoward side-effects that don't undermine its original intent. The literature around sexual abuse (Robohm and Buttenheim 1996) and post-traumatic stress disorder (Menage 1996) indicate that women who have experienced these find vaginal examinations very problematic. Then there is the enlightening paper by Bergstrom *et al*. (1992), still a classic of phenomenological method and of the value of qualitative research. Her video-taping of vaginal examinations in US labour wards revealed the ritual that has evolved around the practice to legitimise such an intrusion into the private space. In essence, she shows the surgical construction of a practice undertaken by strangers that would be totally unacceptable in any other circumstances except in an intimate sexual context between consenting adults. The adoption of a passive patient role and the marked power differential between the patient and the clinician were other taken-for-granted behaviours. More recently, Stewart (2005) came to similar conclusions in a UK-based study. Warren (1999) reminds us that two important questions need asking before any vaginal examination is carried out:

- Why do I need to know this information now?
- Is there any other way I can obtain it?

## Alternative skills for sussing out labour

There is a surprising dearth of any research examining alternatives to vaginal examinations for labour care, given the rich anecdotes that surround this area. Midwives have always taken into account the character of contractions, a woman's response to them and the findings from abdominal palpation. Winter and Duff's chapter in the excellent book, *Childbirth, Midwifery and Concepts of Time* (2010), draws on their masters and doctoral research.

Winter found that independent midwives drew on more holistic cues for getting a 'feel' for labour, like the woman's psychological state and the suitability of the immediate birth environment. Duff tested a labour assessment tool incorporating both physical and observed behaviours and found that experienced midwives tended to classify labours as 'condensed' or 'varied'. Winter and Duff conclude from their research that labour progression is not linear but episodic and idiosyncratic, or 'orderly chaos' as they subtitle their chapter.

Stuart (2000) is possibly unique in relying on abdominal palpation instead of vaginal examination to ascertain progress, and most midwives weigh the results of vaginal examination above contractions and behaviour. However, Stuart states that the degree of descent of the presenting part can be ascertained with the method and there is midwifery anecdote that says undertaking palpation with the woman standing is a more accurate way of determining the descent of the presenting part. Hobbs (1998), among others, advocated the 'purple line' method: a line that runs from the distal margin of the anus up between the buttocks is said to indicate full dilatation when it reaches the natal cleft. Byrne and Edmonds (1990) reported that 89 per cent of women developed the line. Shepherd et al. (2010) found an incidence of 76 per cent in labouring women but significantly did correlation tests with vaginal examination, concluding that there was a medium positive correlation between length of the purple line and cervical dilatation.

Frye (2004), in her extremely comprehensive manual of care during normal birth, writes of monitoring temperature change in the lower leg. As labour progresses so a coldness on touch is noted to move from the ankle up the leg to the knee. Over recent years I have heard from a number of sources of the marker on the forehead of a woman. Possibly originating from traditional birth attendant practices in Peru, this involved feeling for the appearance of a ridge running from between the eyes up to the hairline as labour progresses.

Other wisdom comes from intuitive perceptions that many midwives may recognise but find hard to articulate and even harder to write down, as illustrated by the following story. An experience of intuition was related by home birth midwives who noted in their own bodies the desire to defecate when women they were caring for were approaching full dilatation. Some midwives say they can smell when a labour is progressive. A midwife in Australia's tropical north told me how she used the ebb and flow of the tide to gauge how indigenous island women laboured. They tended to birth at high tide so, as the birthing suite overlooked a tidal bay, she knew they were approaching the second stage of labour when the tide was high. Other anecdotes are around the behaviour of pets and farm animals that seem to know when their owners are labouring. The transitional phase between the first and second stages has been studied by Baker and Kenner (1993), who noted the common vocalisations that mark it.

These are just a few examples of stories that abound in this area. It is an area ripe for observational research but also for articles mapping the richness of midwives' experience. The intuitive hunches of midwives are in danger of being lost as they exist largely as oral stories, not written accounts, possibly because they might be discredited by an evidence orthodoxy that rates empirical verifiability as the standard.

Finally there is the domain of emotional nuance reading that may impact hugely on how labour unfolds (Kennedy *et al.* 2004). I recall one such episode in the birth centre study (Walsh 2006a) when a teenage girl arrived in early labour, very distressed. The midwife asked her mother and sister to leave the room and gently enquired as to how she is. She burst into tears and over the next two hours, the midwife held her in an embrace on a mattress on the floor as the girl sobbed and sobbed. Then she said she was ready and went on to have a normal, rather peaceful birth. In other settings the girl might have been offered an epidural, but this was not pain distress but emotional distress and the skill of the midwife was in her intuitive emotional nuance reading of that and how to bring comfort and support.

## Prolonged labour

The question of what to do when labour is prolonged is a key one if we are to seriously address the epidemic of exogenous oxytocin augmentation. Having extricated ourselves from the straitjacket of progress paradigm, there now exists the possibility of rewriting slow or stalled labour as physiological variation and not pathology. Other options open up now, including simply waiting until labour starts or continuing ongoing support as labour continues more slowly.

Simkin and Ancheta's little gem, *The Labour Progress Handbook* (2011), promotes options other than the traditional medical approaches of artificial rupture of membranes (ARM) and oxytocin augmentation in a much more holistic orientation to labour care. They take us through a series of postural and positional options that may stimulate the labour and a number of accompanying comfort/support measures like the application of hot towels to the lower back. Research supports their focus on movement as Lawrence *et al.*'s (2009) review showed in shortened labour. Simkin and Ancheta's book includes a taxonomy of possible causes of slow labour and appropriate interventions, and at the end of the list of interventions are medical ones to be considered when all other possibilities have been exhausted.

Anderson (2004) adds to the slow labour debate by citing organisational 'dystocias' that may impact on the labouring women. These may include:

- lack of continuity of care and continuous support by midwives 'dystocia';
- inexperienced doctors at the start of their rotation 'dystocia';
- absence of expertise during the summer holidays, weekends, night shifts, bank holidays 'dystocia';
- disagreements between midwife and obstetrician 'dystocia';
- inadequate handovers because of fatigue or intimidation 'dystocia'.

Clearly these are usually not considered when women's labours are deemed to be 'failing to progress' but they may well be contextually relevant.

Cluett et al.'s (2004) fascinating paper on the advantage of hydrotherapy over an oxytocin infusion in nulliparous women with prolonged labour appears to have had little impact in maternity hospitals, at least in the UK. The research showed those women who entered birthing pools when their labour slowed ultimately received less augmentation (71 per cent versus 96 per cent) and fewer epidurals (47 per cent versus 66 per cent) than those who were medically managed with syntocinon. Since then, Zanetti-Dällenbach et al.'s (2006) paper has concluded that water immersion shortens labour length. These findings suggest that every labour ward should have, alongside the sundry ampoules of oxytocin and packs of disposable amnihooks, birthing pools available. They are, after all, the more effective and safer option and one resonant with normal physiology.

As already mentioned, encouraging mobility and posture change also shortens labour. A number of complementary therapies are starting to demonstrate an evidence base around shortening labour which indicates a possible role in prolonged labour. These include acupuncture (Skilnand et al. 2002), acupressure (Kyeong et al. 2004), hypnosis (Harmon et al. 1990), yoga (Chuntharapat et al. 2008) and massage (Field et al. 1997). In addition there is a physiological rationale and tentative evidence that nipple stimulation may be beneficial (Razgaitis and Lyvers 2010).

For the small number of women who have a pathological prolonged labour due to a position problem or the poorly defined 'incordinate uterine contractions', then ARM has for decades been the first option for medical management. However, Smyth et al.'s (2008) fairly recently updated review now concludes that ARM does not shorten labour, even in nulliparous women, and may contribute to a higher caesarean section rate. This overturns decades of conventional wisdom and thus far these findings have not impacted on practice. Clearly more research is needed, though ARM has been subjected to plenty so far. The other recourse is oxytocin augmentation, though this is usually prescribed after ARM. There is uncertainty over its effectiveness in achieving a spontaneous vaginal birth, with Bugg *et al.* (2006) concluding it only does this in 51 per cent of women diagnosed with dystocia. There is also debate over whether early or late recourse to oxytocin augmentation improves the rates of spontaneous birth (Wei *et al.* 2009, Dencker *et al.* 2009, Hinshaw *et al.* 2008). What there is not much doubt about are exogenous oxytocin's propensity to hyperstimulate the uterus and the link between it and poor neonatal outcome (Oscarsson *et al.* 2006). For this reason the American College of Obstetricians advise titrating it very carefully against uterine actions and only using the minimum amount possible to establish and advance labour (Clark *et al.* 2009).

In summary, the diagnosis of dystocia is poorly delineated and understood. It needs decoupling from labour plateaus where the uterus is just resting and from the latent phase that can extend to 5–6 cm dilatation. Then a group remains that may have a positional problem, those with ill-defined incoordinate uterine contractions and those that have a true dystocia for whom an oxytocin infusion will not be effective. Recent research into lactic acid levels in women with prolonged labour may help distinguish those likely to respond to oxytocin and those who will not (Wiberg-Itzel *et al.* 2008). What can be concluded with some confidence is that dystocia is probably over-diagnosed and over-treated in models of care across the Western world.

## 'Being with' not 'doing to' labouring women

The quest to dismantle assembly-line birth, removing women from the intrapartum time line and rehabilitating belief in 'unique normality' of labour for individual women challenges us to radically rethink our focus and orientation to normal labour care. Hints of a different way of situating ourselves with women are in the writings of midwives and they speak in paradox and metaphor. Leap (2000b) tells of 'the less we do, the more we give' and Kennedy (2000) of 'doing nothing well' in her insightful study of expert US midwives. Fahy (1998) conceptualises the work of the midwife as 'being with' women, not 'doing to' them, and Anderson (2004) quips that good labour care requires the midwife 'to drink tea intelligently'. All these writers are alluding not to a temporally regulated activity marked by task completions but to a disposition towards compassionate companionship with women that is a 'masterly inactivity' (RCM 2006). As a birth centre midwife offered during an interview: 'it's about being comfortable when there is nothing to do.' All of this is summed up beautifully in Browne and Chandra's (2009) thoughtful paper calling for a new movement – 'slow midwifery' – which allows for the power of 'presence' (Kennedy *et al.* 2010) to manifest.

These ideas are counter-cultural in an environment heavily inscribed with a 'doing' ethos as maternity hospitals are and also anathema for the medical model where there is a 'compulsion to act' (Grol and Grimshaw 2003). It is challenging in a resource-tight health service where time and motion analysis are skewed to activity measurement. Yet Enkin *et al.* (2000), as already mentioned in Chapter 1, the doyens of evidence-based maternity care, understood the truism that sometimes 'what really counts, cannot be counted' and I suggest that supportive labour care fits precisely into this category.

## Conclusion

Labour care urgently needs to adjust to a new paradigm of 'labour rhythms' instead of 'labour progress' for normal childbirth. This endeavour will require a reorienting of thinking to incorporate greater flexibility in how labour unfolds for different women, both in how it starts and how it continues. A greater focus on the birth environment and on the role of birth companions is also required so that the hormonal cascade of birth can be optimally facilitated. The special task for midwives is, in partnership with women, to discover and nourish their personal template of labour rhythms. This is not so much a task as a disposition to 'being with' women as a compassionate companion for the labour journey.

All of the above requires the deinstitutionalising of labour care, in particular the dismantling of the childbirth assembly-line that regulates primarily not for clinical ends but for an organisational imperative. A twinned approach with both clinical and organisational revisioning is required for the contextual bind maternity services have managed to evolve over the past fifty years. Only then will the dance of labour re-emerge in all its heterogeneous beauty.

## Practice recommendations

- Maternity services need to prioritise the creation of a suitable environmental and social ambience for individual women.
- Services should facilitate women in early labour either staying at home, going to a birth centre or attending a triage facility (avoid labour wards if at all possible).
- Time variations in labour could be understood as differing rhythms for different women, not as potential pathology, unless the uterus is working hard and there is no progress.

- Services should facilitate midwives acquiring skills in recognising labour rhythms, including developing their intuition.
- If partograms are used:

  1 then a four-hour action line is a useful marker for recognising prolonged labour
  2 with a minimal cervical dilatation rate of 0.5 cm/hour.

- Care for prolonged labour should prioritise physiological/psychological/social support before medical interventions.
- Practices around the use of ARM need reviewing in the light of evidence challenging its effectiveness.
- Exogenous oxytocin should be reserved for dystocia that does not respond to any other intervention and then used sparingly.
- Services should review their use of vaginal examinations in labour in the light of these recommendations.

## Questions for reflection

How might you go about addressing the shift from 'labour progress' mindset to a 'labour rhythms' approach?

What should be done about the practice of repeated vaginal examinations in labour?

How could the use of intuition in 'sussing out labour rhythms' be encouraged?

How might you develop a holistic approach to 'slow labour'?

What options have you got where you work around care of women in early labour and can they be improved?

What steps can you take to optimise birth environment and social ambience for the labouring women you care for?

# Chapter 5    **Fetal heart monitoring in labour**

- Current evidence base of electronic fetal monitoring (EFM)
- Fetal mortality and morbidity related to birth asphyxia
- Alternative technologies for assessing fetal well-being
- Conclusion
- Practice recommendations
- Questions for reflection

Continuous cardiotocography (CTG) encapsulates many of the issues that distinguish the social model from the biomedical model of care: our relationship with birth technologies, the interpretation of equivocal evidence, notions of risk and the significance of the birth environment. All of these need exploring in the context of fetal monitoring. As I practise in a large maternity hospital I experience exactly the same concerns regarding fetal monitoring now as I did when I was first prompted to write on this area in 1998. Since then I have had the opportunity to experience more births at home and in birth centres and these have informed my present views. One thing that is striking about environments where intermittent auscultation is used is how rarely fetal distress is diagnosed, when on large labour wards it is a common occurrence. This is not explained solely by the different case mixes of each setting.

In this chapter I will explore the evidence base of different types of fetal monitoring. I will engage with the risk/benefit ratio in attempting to apply the research findings. This requires us to examine the iatrogenic effects of continuous CTG. The discussion needs to scope the issue of perinatal death and injury and their relationship to intrapartum events. We will briefly examine competing or adjunct technologies to see whether they help our deliberations. The role of technology in modern birth practice will be discussed and how that impacts on childbirth attendants and birthing women. Finally, the ubiquity of risk needs addressing if we are to challenge powerful discourses that shape attitudes and practices towards fetal monitoring on the ground.

Continuous CTG has always been a provocative area of intrapartum practice to examine because strong custom and practice routines preceded robust evidence. The technology was widespread and embedded in practice before the randomised controlled trials (RCTs) appeared. The RCTs, summarised in Alfirevic *et al.*'s (2006) review, challenge the embedded practice, not only casting doubt over its use for low-risk women but failing to show any perinatal mortality benefit for high-risk women as well. Over the past couple of years, critiques of evidence-based health care have exposed the possibility of biases in research reporting and implantation, with technological innovations receiving favourable evaluations (de Vries and Lemmens 2006). It is therefore fascinating to observe the impact of negative findings from the evaluation of a technology. Authoritative voices like the National Institute for Clinical Excellence (NICE) in the UK and the national colleges of obstetricians in the USA and Australia have thrown their weight behind judicious application of continuous CTG so that more maternity services are now complying with evidence recommendations.

## Current evidence base of electronic fetal monitoring (EFM)

The updated systematic review is a very interesting read (Alfirevic *et al.* 2006). As well as undertaking a new meta-analysis, the background and discussion sections seek to explore contextual issues related to continuous CTG, which are often neglected in systematic reviews. Under possible disadvantages of CTG, they write: '[it] shifts staff focus and resources away from the mother and may encourage a belief that all perinatal mortality and neurological injury can be prevented' (p. 4). They also comment on the small amount of qualitative work done on women's views and experiences, though they miss a paper on the impact of continuous CTG on midwives (Hindley *et al.* 2006). More recently, Greer (2010) has written eloquently about the powerful social norms operationalised around EFM's use on labour suites and their constraining impact on midwifery decision-making. Understanding these subtleties is so important in addressing barriers to the implementation of evidence.

Alfirevic *et al.* (2006) include twelve trials involving 37,000 women in total. Compared to intermittent auscultation, continuous CTG showed no significant difference in perinatal death but was associated with a halving of neonatal seizures, although no significant difference was detected in cerebral palsy. There was a significant increase in caesarean sections and assisted vaginal births in the continuous CTG group. There were no differences between the two groups in relation to Apgar scores, neonatal admissions or hypoxic ischaemic encephalopathy.

In discussing the findings on seizures, the authors urge caution in interpreting what this means in the long term. Though there was no increase in cerebral palsy or ischaemic encephalopathy, the absence of long-term follow-up of the cohort does not exclude the possibility that they may have more minor neurological sequelae. Using numbers needed to treat method, one neonatal seizure might be prevented in every 660 cases if all women were continuously monitored. This has to be balanced against the much greater risk of emergency caesarean section (one in every fifty-eight women).

The results of the systematic reviews have shaped national and local guidelines in this area which pretty universally recommend continuous CTG for high-risk groups. Even here, it needs to be recognised that this is a pragmatic and common-sense 'take' on the evidence which does not show any difference in perinatal death and cerebral palsy even in high-risk groups. Ironically, one trial that compared intermittent with continuous fetal monitoring in preterm labours found higher rates of cerebral palsy in the latter group (Luthy *et al.* 1987) and the only other study that examined the two methods in high-risk women showed no differences in outcome (Herbst and Ingemarsson 1994).

There is anecdotal evidence that some maternity units allow intermittent auscultation in particular groups such as induction of labours that don't require syntocinon. Madaan and Trivedi (2006) undertook an RCT of the two methods in women who had previous caesarean sections and found a higher vaginal birth rate in the intermittent group and higher rate of caesarean section for non-reassuring CTG in the continuously monitored group without any impact on perinatal outcome.

If continuous CTG is an imperfect technology, then it makes no sense at all to install the very expensive central bank monitoring system where individual women's traces can be viewed centrally. Yet many labour wards across the world have invested in this technology. It is not surprising to find that the evaluations of these monitoring systems showed no improvement in fetal outcome but a probable rise in caesarean section (Withiam-Leitch *et al.* 2006).

## Fetal mortality and morbidity related to birth asphyxia

There are a number of drivers for the high priority given to fetal heart surveillance during intrapartum care, among them the desire to reduce intrapartum-related perinatal deaths and cerebral palsy, compliance with the Clinical Negligence Scheme for Trusts (CNST) standards, the discourse of risk and an optimistic notion of birth technology.

### *Perinatal mortality*

Though the systematic review did not show any difference in perinatal mortality, the authors rightly argue that, because of the rarity of this outcome, to reduce deaths by 1 in 1000, 50,000 women would have to be randomised. Such a huge trail will never be mounted. These numbers are required because deaths related to intrapartum asphyxia represent less than 0.1 per cent of total deaths (Stewart *et al.* 1998). Within this category, there will be sentinel hypoxic events like cord prolapse and placental abruption that relate to sudden death. Chronic asphyxia leading to fetal demise is rare indeed. Alfirevic and colleagues argue that morbidity outcomes are better targeted, specifically cerebral palsy which generates huge liabilities for maternity units if negligence is proved.

### *Perinatal morbidity*

However, the relationship between cerebral palsy and intrapartum asphyxia is equally as problematic. The reported incidence of cerebral palsy in the

Western world is between 0.1 per cent and 0.2 per cent (MacDonald 1996, Nelson *et al.* 1996) but of these incidences only 10–20 per cent are thought to be related to intrapartum events (Scheller and Nelson 1994). The remainder, MacDonald (1996) reminds us, were made up of a 90 per cent group whose cerebral palsy was related to some antenatal insult and a 10 per cent group where it was caused by pathologic events after the birth. Clearly the antenatal period is where the focus of concern should be directed, not the intrapartum. Within the 10–20 per cent group some, like the perinatal deaths, will be linked to an acute hypoxic episode.

In addition, the related precursor condition severe hypoxic ischaemic encephalopathy (HIE), more accurately known as hypoxic encephalopathy, has an incidence of about 2.5 per cent in term infants (Graham *et al.* 2008). In other words, in a hospital of 6000 births, there will be 12–14 cases per year. Similar to cerebral palsy, only about 15 per cent of these are related to intrapartum events as the vast majority are known to be linked to antenatal causation (Graham *et al.* 2008). Thus, out of 12–14 cases in a 6000-birth hospital, about two cases will be related to intrapartum events.

Relating the tiny number of intrapartum-related HIE and cerebral palsy cases to abnormal findings on a fetal heart trace is asking a lot of a flawed technology. The relative ineffectiveness of continuous CTG to achieve this has frustrated many maternity care professionals. How is it that a 'real-time' trace is not able to discriminate between babies who are compromised and those who are not? The problem rests with continuous CTG's sensitivity and specificity as a screening and diagnostic test.

Hillan's (1991) paper remains the best explanation for those of us without epidemiological training. It succinctly explains these terms. The continuous CTG is characterised by a relatively high sensitivity (the ability to identify those fetuses that are distressed) and a low specificity (the ability to identify those that aren't). It therefore has a high false positive rate, i.e. it identifies many babies with abnormal traces who are not actually distressed. This high false positive rate has plagued clinicians and researchers alike since evaluations started in the 1970s, because the operative and assisted delivery rates skyrocketed without any demonstrable impact on perinatal mortality or morbidity rates. An increase in caesarean section rates of up to 160 per cent have been recorded in some studies (Haverkamp *et al.* 1976) and an increase of up to 30 per cent in assisted vaginal birth rates (MacDonald *et al.* 1985). These figures have decreased somewhat since then but are probably still too high. Taking the specific example of multiple late decelerations and decreased variability, ominous signs on a CTG, these features have a false positive rate of 99.8 per cent (Nelson *et al.* 1996). In other words, the vast majority of babies demonstrating these patterns are healthy and well.

### Litigious environment

Our adversarial legal system which requires the establishment of negligence before a family can obtain adequate financial help to care for a profoundly disabled child has spawned an elaborate protective mechanism for hospitals and health departments. In the UK, a scheme (Clinical Negligence Scheme for Trusts) that indemnifies these institutions for claims requires prescriptive standards to be met (CNST 2011). A number of these standards pertain to fetal monitoring. Fetal monitoring has become central to litigation because cerebral palsy claims, when focusing on preventable aspects of damage, home in on intrapartum care. The CTG becomes crucial evidence. What is paradoxical here is that we have already established that the technology is imperfect and that cerebral palsy is largely a morbidity related to the antenatal period, yet legal cases seem to regularly find fault with care around fetal monitoring. A further irony is that the expert opinions sought to establish negligence are from obstetricians and midwives who should be familiar with the problematic evidence base of continuous CTG, though Kesselheim and Studdert's (2006) recent paper suggests otherwise. Their examination of the profile of expert witnesses raised concerns over their level of knowledge. The distorting effect of hindsight bias (Zain *et al.* 1998) adds to the problematic nature of this whole process. Hindsight bias is the understandable human failing of over-optimistically assuming clinician failure in a case review that the reviewer knows the outcome of in advance.

CNST requires mandatory six-monthly training on continuous CTG for all staff involved in intrapartum care. This standard reinforces the distorted view that it is practitioners' flawed interpretation, not the technology itself, which is at fault. It also feeds the impression we are warned of by Alfirevic *et al.* (2006) that undue focus on the CTG 'encourages a belief that all perinatal mortality and neurological injury can be prevented'.

A move to a no-fault compensation scheme for perinatal injury would be a very welcome development, not just to address the disproportionate dominance of fetal monitoring in labour care but as a more humane mechanism for dealing with the personal pain for both client and plaintiff of the current adversarial system. The pain and distress was powerfully and graphically illustrated at the third International Normal Birth Conference when the story of an intrapartum litigation case was courageously acted out by the actual participants and has now been published (Byrom, Murray *et al.* 2010)

### Risk

A discourse of risk feeds litigation and is ubiquitous in contemporary maternity care. Risk fits comfortably within the biomedical model of childbirth with its 'only normal in retrospect' mindset. It sows the fallacy that uncertainty can be eliminated from seminal life events if they are kept under surveillance by experts. This has never been true of childbirth and never will be. Recent thinking on risk has endorsed the phrase 'risk acceptance' (Walsh 2006c) to acknowledge this truism. Instead of medically scrutinising all births, a more effective approach would be to predicate care delivery on models known to be efficacious: one-to-one support in labour, continuity of carer, choice and care that empowers women – these all have a sound evidence base as elaborated on in Chapter 2. Risk's power to dictate emotions in the birth room are illustrated by equivocal CTG tracing. The following story reveals this power.

A father relates the story of his first son's birth. Suspected fetal distress was an ongoing concern throughout the labour, with various doctors and midwives adopting a 'wait and see' approach. Little of this was communicated to the parents and the information that was given was equivocal, as often the interpretation of CTG is. Both parents picked up on the anxiety of the midwife. Uncertainty persisted until in late second stage a forceps delivery was carried out for suspected fetal distress. The baby was born in good condition and there was relief all round but for the father it was the most terrifying experience of his life. He thought his child would be born brain-damaged.

Greer (2010) and Lankshear *et al.*'s (2005) analysis of decision-making around CTG use on labour wards illustrate how CTG interpretation provokes uncertainty and fear, which has the effect of undermining women's autonomy. For a broader sweep on the impact of the risk discourse on maternity care, see MacKenzie and van Teijlingen (2010).

### *Role of technology*

Technologies seldom work in a linear way as a panacea for a specific problem. Though they are developed for benefit, commonly they have unintended consequences. Iatrogenic effects are significant with continuous CTG and include all the complications of emergency caesarean sections. The following is not an exhaustive list: infection (van Ham *et al.* 1997); haemorrhage, pain and immobility; placenta praevia in subsequent pregnancy (Ananth *et al.* 1997); reduced subsequent fertility; repeat caesarean section for next pregnancy (Hemminki 1996); post-traumatic stress syndrome (Ryding *et al.* 1998); and reduced breastfeeding (DiMatteo *et al.* 1996). In addition, more assisted vaginal births, another iatrogenic effect of continuous CTG, result in more urinary stress incontinence (Arya *et al.* 2001), more anal sphincter tears (MacArthur *et al.* 2005) and more dyspareunia (Bick *et al.* 2008).

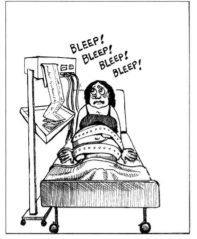
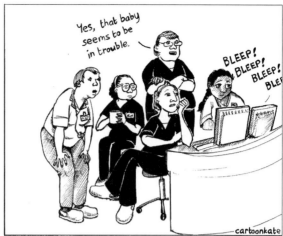

Technologies are not value-neutral. They are indicative of a techno-rational paradigm that supervalues technological innovation (Lauritzen and Sachs 2001). This has significant implications for labour and birth because the use of technologies in this context can undermine both normal physiology and the dynamics of birth room relationships. Women have hinted at this in evaluations of their experience of CTG, stating that it constricted their movements and, more tellingly, distracted midwives from focusing on their needs (Munro *et al.* 2004). McKay's (1991) fascinating paper develops this idea in her interviews of women who had been continuously monitored. Women felt redundant as a source of information and felt marginalised from their carers who spent much of their time watching the trace. She drew diagrams of the layout of the birth room to illustrate lines of sight between the midwife, the woman and her partner. All were positioned so that the monitor formed the apex of all their attentions. McKay uses the words 'dehumanised' and 'alienating' in a forceful indictment of the technology usurping the person as the primary focus. There is a sense that a midwife has a kind of relationship with a monitor. It communicates on two levels, visual and auditory, and dictates priorities of care when the tracing is suboptimal.

In the only examination to date of midwives' views, Munro *et al.* (2002) also found that continuous CTG interfered with the relationship between midwives and women and was often the starting point of a cascade of intervention. Midwives spoke of juxtaposing elements: the CTG as a tool of reassurance and as an instrument of anxiety.

Further problems for continuous CTG are both intra- and inter-observer reliability (Devane and Lalor 2005). Educational packages and algorithms have been developed to address these but there is no evidence so far that they have been successful (Hindley *et al.* 2005).

## Alternative technologies for assessing fetal well-being

Fetal blood sampling has been widely adopted on labour wards to improve the sensitivity of continuous CTG and Thacker et al.'s (2006) previous review recommended its use. The new review (Alfirevic et al. 2006) no longer endorses it, finding it did not contribute to lower caesarean rates.

A variety of other technologies are currently being studied as an alternative or as an adjunct to continuous CTG. The most promising is the fetal ECG. Neilson's (2006) Cochrane review found this may be useful for women with non-reassuring CTG patterns. It has the disadvantage of requiring the membranes to be ruptured. In Sweden, where one of the original trials was held and where experience with the so-called STAN monitors is extensive, Noren et al.'s (2006) observational study concluded that its use did appear to show a reduction in fetal metabolic acidosis. There is some evidence that fetal pulse oximetry measurement is as good as (Allen et al. 2004) or better than fetal blood sampling in discriminating abnormal CTG patterns (Salamalekis et al. 2006). Fetal lactate measurement is also under review and showing some promise (Gjerris et al. 2008). Finally, so-called smart monitors that assist in CTG analysis have had some initial evaluation (Schiermeier et al. 2008) and are now the subject of a very expensive multi-centre trail (INFANT) (NPEU 2010).

On a related topic, three admission test RCTs have been systematically reviewed by Blix et al. (2005) and found to increase epidural, continuous CTG and fetal blood sampling rates in labour without bestowing any fetal benefit.

## Conclusion

In millions of labours across the world, babies are being continuously monitored without sound evidence of overall benefit. A trade-off between reducing neonatal seizures, though there is no evidence of long-term complications from these, and many more women having effectively unnecessary caesarean sections has been made. Continuous CTG has become the most common of obstetric technologies and the centre of attention in a birthing milieu dominated by risk and fear of litigation. It is perhaps the ultimate expression of Foucault's (1973) panopticism (the institutional gaze) in the childbirth context. Though its surveillance is directed at the fetus, it effectively controls the woman by restricting her movement and surrounding her with an atmosphere of latent anxiety. It controls the midwife by monopolising her attention, distracting her from being wholly present to the woman in other ways. As a technology, it exemplifies a concern expressed by Downs (1966) almost fifty years ago: 'gains in technology seem to be resulting in the loss of human essence.' It is important to remember that the healthy term fetus must be exposed to the stress of labour to prepare itself for extra-uterine transition, as Harrison's (1999) important paper points out. Intermittent auscultation is cheap and non-invasive. Critically it does not distract the woman or the midwife from tuning into each other and to the subtleties and power of the labour. I suspect this synchronicity may actually be much more significant for the health of the baby than the reactive preoccupation with a strip of paper.

## Practice recommendations

- Abandon continuous CTG during normal labour and birth.
- Don't do admission traces on women anticipating a normal labour.
- Separate normal birth facilities from high-risk delivery suites.
- Remove all electronic fetal monitors from normal birth areas.
- Consider the impact that continuous CTG may have on midwives' relationships with women in labour.
- Consider the impact that continuous CTG may have on women's experience of labour and birth.

---

### Questions for reflection

Could you stimulate a debate about the appropriateness of continuous CTG and its impact on the dynamics of the birth environment where you work?

How can risk, litigation and fetal monitoring positively contribute to supporting normal birth?

How might you stimulate a wider discussion of the role of technology in normal birth?

---

# Chapter 6   **Mobility and posture in labour**

Progress towards maximising mobility in labour and the adoption of upright posture for birth has been very slow over the past ten years. A national survey of UK maternity units made for depressing reading in this area: 88 per cent of all births occurred on beds and 79 per cent of all birth postures were either sitting or lying (Redshaw *et al.* 2006). The situation in the USA was slightly better with 57 per cent of women surveyed stating they gave birth on a bed in a lying position (Declerq *et al.* 2006). Alongside these figures sit audit data from small midwifery-led units where upright birth posture rates are around 80 per cent (ISIS 2006) and beds are conspicuous by their absence from birth rooms.

The type and amount of evidence in this area provides compelling evidence for the value of mobility in the first stage of labour and for the adoption of upright birth postures in the second stage of labour. Gupta and Hofmeyr (2006) refer to the different types of evidence sources in their preamble to the current Cochrane review on position for birth when they mention early anthropological studies of indigenous peoples who, it is documented, favoured upright posture for giving birth (Jarcho 1934). Kitzinger (2000), in her beautiful book *Rediscovering Birth*, devotes an entire chapter to this facet of current indigenous practices in varying places of the world, while Coppen's (2005) important book covers the history of childbirth posture in some detail and is an excellent reference for those seeking more detail.

It is very rare to see positive comments made about historical birth practices in clinical journals where a certain imperialistic arrogance usually discredits them. However, Lavin and McGregor (1992) tell us in the *Journal of Feto-Maternal Medicine* that contemporary birth care can learn from northern Native American Indians. They go on to describe the technique of the supported squat using a sling hung from above. Balaskas (1995) draws on archaeological evidence from artefacts, cave drawing and writings to reveal the mainstream nature of upright birth in ancient Egyptian, Greek and Roman civilisations.

All of these sources pose important questions for contemporary birthing practices. Has the physiology of birth changed so much that these sources have nothing worthwhile to say to us today? Or are they communicating a deep and profound wisdom about birth that we ignore at our peril? At one level, thousands of years of tradition and cross-cultural congruence/consensus on birth posture seems to be far more convincing than fewer than ten research studies spread over the last thirty years. In fact, I am inclined to use these alternative sources of evidence as my touchstone for best evidence in this area and the research studies as adjuncts and confirmatory.

Some of my antipathy to research in this area arises from the history of birth posture over the past 300 years, in particular, its medicalisation in westernised countries. One of the earliest written records of women being required to lie down for birth is from Mauriceau's textbook of 1678 (Dunn 1991). But it was the invention of the forceps which established that ubiquitous symbol of modern childbirth, the bed, as central to parturition (Boyle 2000). In so doing, it reversed an ancient maxim that *childbirth attendants should fit around the woman* so that now the mother took up a position to facilitate the ease of the attendant in delivering the baby. If you asked a group of women to brainstorm for fifteen minutes the worst possible birth position, they may well come up with the lithotomy. Yet this became mainstream for not just assisted vaginal birth but also for normal birth.

The introduction of anaesthesia and narcotics confirmed the centrality of the bed for birth, for now women were not safe to mobilise as either their conscious level or motor strength was impaired. The semi-recumbent posture, though adopted at the beginning of the second stage, would often become supine by the time of birth as women slipped down the bed in the pushing phase. By the 1980s and the hospitalisation of most birth in the Western world, the dangers of supine hypotension syndrome for late pregnancy and labour were well known and labour suites addressed this problem by the utilisation of soft wedges to tip labouring women off their backs. As student midwives of this time, many of us thought this was a curious way to address a problem that was

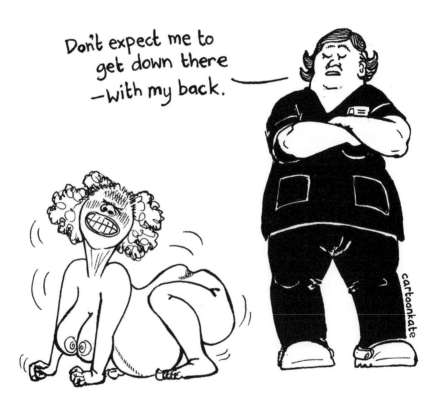

all about birth room furniture. Our strategy of getting women off beds or even removing beds from the birth room were not even in the frame for consideration, so steeped was the birthing culture at the time in managed birth.

During the 1970s, Caldeyro-Barcia, working in South America, conducted his famous physiological studies revealing the disadvantages of supine postures for labour and birth, particularly for the fetus (Caldeyro-Barcia 1979). It is surprising, therefore, to find that the later studies of mobilisation during labour and of the birth posture all tested the 'experimental' interventions of freedom of movement or upright birth posture compared with the standard, 'normative' practice of remaining supine on the bed. It shows how far we had moved from Enkin's fundamental tenet that any intervention should display advantage over normal birth physiology before being routinely introduced. In these trials we have the paradox of physiological behaviours needing to prove advantage over the clearly inferior managed birth model.

## Mobility in the first stage of labour

A number of trials of mobility during labour have concluded that it reduces the need for analgesics, shortens labour and improves satisfaction with care (Bloom et al. 1998, MacLennan et al. 1994, Hemminki and Saarikoski 1983). Early studies noted trends in favour of mobility, rather than statistically significant differences, in the following areas: stronger uterine contractility, shorter labour, less augmentation, fewer operative deliveries, less fetal distress (Flynn et al. 1978, Read et al. 1981, Albers et al. 1997). A closer look at the trials reveals that, in some of the studies, women in the experimental arm were exposed to other birth interventions like EFM, ARM and frequent vaginal examinations, and yet the value of mobility still expressed itself. This suggests that the drive to be mobile or to change position is so powerful it can overcome these restrictions.

In 2009, Lawrence et al. systematically reviewed all the RCTs on maternal positions and mobility in the first stage of labour and concluded that mobility reduced the length of the first stage of labour and reduced epidural rates. Mobility and upright posture were not associated with any adverse outcomes. Disappointingly, they then advocated the rather weak position that women should be encouraged to adopt whatever position was comfortable during the first stage, rather than advising of the benefits of mobility and upright posture and encouraging their adoption.

The desire to be mobile in labour is impinged upon by the environment, both in the physical space and in the degree of privacy. In the home birth setting, both of these issues are easily addressed but in institutional settings they are a challenge. Many free-standing midwifery units (FMUs) address these areas by being situated on ground floors where there is often access to outside gardens and where the smallness of scale means reduced 'traffic' through the centre. There may well be a sense of 'grounding' that is significant for human childbirth. This is, of course, lost in institutional birth where women are rarely labouring on the ground floor. Connectedness to the earth could be subliminally reassuring for both the woman and her birth companions. It is the necessity for privacy that is so undermined by institutional birth. Women cannot roam, disrobe or vocalise with ease as everywhere outside their room is public space. Indigenous birth teaches us much about the guarding of the birth space (Kitzinger 2000) and recent studies of the importance of women having control over their responses to labour (Carter 2010) resonate with this. Women need to feel free to express themselves – a freedom that requires guarantees of privacy.

Earlier I have written of the 'dance of labour' in reference to the chemistry of birth hormones (see Chapter 4) but the metaphor is literal in respect of women's movements in labour. Many will sway and swivel in rhythm with their contractions and it is no surprise that bellydancing is being taught during pregnancy in some parts of the world (www.visionarydance.com/birthdanceB.html). Simkin and Ancheta (2011) devote whole chapters in their book on labour progress to postures and positions, seeing it as fundamental to labour rhythms and to the act of birthing.

It is reasonable to conclude from this body of work that any intervention that physically inhibits regular positional change, shackles women to beds or psychologically discourages them from moving is going to be undermining of birth physiology. The benefits of interventions like EFM have to be weighed against these counter-productive effects and every effort made to accommodate the woman's changes of posture by adjusting belts and leads. The advent of wireless CTG monitors has helped in this area. The same applies to intravenous lines. If the bed is undermining this freedom of movement, then it should be either removed or pushed against a wall so that a woman has fuller access to room space. This is an area where much greater flexibility could exist than is currently practised on many labour wards (Spiby *et al.* 2003). The default position of the bed is so easily assumed when women have other co-existent interventions. However, there are stories out there of women giving birth on the floor or in a variety of upright postures while attached to monitors or drips, and they represent some of the most inventive midwifery practices around, reclaiming normality.

Specifically in relation to rotating malpositions (lateral and posterior) in late pregnancy or during the first stage of labour, the adoption of a knee/chest position has been studied in a few trials and showed that, though backache was relieved, there was no reduction in the incidence of malpositions (Hunter *et al.* 2007).

## Posture in the second stage of labour

Before discussing the detail of actual giving birth postures, I want to make some observations about positions in the second stage of labour. There is some debate about what constitutes upright or supine postures for birth. If a woman is reclining at less than 45 per cent to the horizontal, then she is clearly more lying than sitting and her position is recumbent. If the second stage commences sitting up on a bed, then by the time of birth, the slippage down the bed during pushing probably means she has dipped under the 45 per cent threshold. For this reason I class conventional bed postures as recumbent in the main, unless the bed has been adapted to promote more upright sitting. Of course a variety of non-back positions can be taken up on the bed, like kneeling, all-fours and side-lying. Lateral postures are often classed as variants of upright, though clearly the gravity effect is not as pronounced. In summary, I would class recumbent postures as supine, lithotomy, semi-recumbent less than 45 per cent to the horizontal and McRoberts, while in upright postures I would include squatting, kneeling, standing, sitting greater than 45 per cent, lateral, all-fours and variants of these.

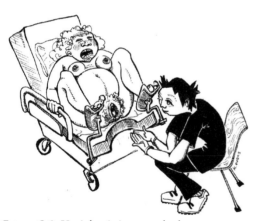

FIGURE 6.1 Upright sitting on a bed.

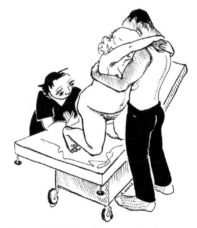

FIGURE 6.2 Kneeling on a bed.

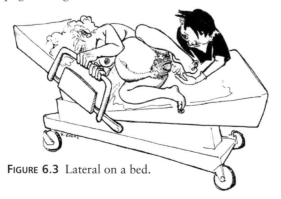

FIGURE 6.3 Lateral on a bed.

There is little doubt that midwives themselves profoundly influence the choices women make regarding birth posture (De Jonge and Lagro-Janssen 2004). It is likely that midwives' advice to women is influenced by their competence at assisting birth in non-recumbent positions. One of De Jonge and Lagro-Janssen's findings was that undertaking a vaginal examination in the second stage appeared to be linked to a semi-recumbent birth because women stayed in the recumbent posture after the examination. They suggest withholding the procedure unless there is some clinical concern. Flint (1986) in her seminal book, *Sensitive Midwifery*, went further by advocating carrying out vaginal exams in whatever position the woman was in, even if this meant doing them from a posterior approach. Her diagrams showed how this altered what was being felt and how to diagnose fetal position 'upside down'. Twenty years on the rationale for any exams during the second stage require robust justification but Flint's principle, reprising the ancient dictum to fit around the woman, rather than her fitting around the attendant, still applies.

There is a sense in which posture impacts on attitude and we are indebted to Balaskas (1995) for alerting us to the implications of this. Her 'stranded beetle' metaphor graphically captures the psychosocial dimensions of birth posture to illustrate the powerlessness and helplessness of being on your back. In this position, the woman is passive as she assumes the pose of a compliant 'patient' and her status vis-à-vis her professional carer is subordinate. Spatial dynamics are disrupted if the woman is upright, or on the floor. Her marked territory, even in a hospital setting, is greater than the confines of the bed. She is either at the attendant's level or the attendant must get low to the floor to communicate with her. These are subtle alterations but they do suggest greater independence, self-direction and control for the woman and the corollary of the midwife adjusting, giving way, shifting the initiative to the woman.

De Jonge *et al.* (2004) and Gupta *et al.* (2004) have both done meta-analyses of positions for giving birth and conclude a number of advantages for upright posture:

- shorter second stage
- fewer episiotomies
- fewer assisted births
- less severe pain
- bearing down easier
- fewer fetal heart abnormalities.

The only outcome that favoured supine posture was a reduced blood loss (<500 ml), though this may have been related to the fact that measurement of blood loss is more accurate in upright posture. Terry *et al.*'s (2006) non-randomised clinical trial concurred with these results, though they concluded that blood loss and vulval oedema were less in upright posture. Finally Ragnar *et al.*'s (2006) trial which compared sitting and kneeling birth positions found women preferred kneeling and they experienced less pain that way.

From an evidence perspective, there are other factors that need mentioning that show physiological and anatomical advantages for upright position. Clearly gravity is working for you, possibly contributing to women saying that bearing down was easier. Gravity is an example of common-sense evidence that does not need an RCT. From time to time, common sense needs to be invoked in intrapartum care to argue against unnecessary evaluations of something that has obvious benefits. For example, do we need an RCT of maintaining privacy, of relating respectfully and of the need to listen to women during labour? These aspects come under treating an individual with dignity and caring for women with compassion and sensitivity.

The avoidance of supine hypotension syndrome has clear physiological benefit for the fetus (Johnstone *et al.* 1987), which is almost certainly reflected in fewer fetal heart abnormalities. In upright postures the flexion and abduction of the hips, combined with the freedom for the coccyx to articulate backwards, provide greater room at the pelvic outlet, both in the anterior/posterior and transverse dimensions (Michel *et al.* 2002). Essentially when the pelvis is not resting on anything and occupies free space, the diameters of the outlet will be maximised. All of these factors contribute to another clear finding from systematic reviews – women prefer upright postures, especially if they have previously used them (De Jonge and Lagro-Janssen 2004).

Given the overwhelming evidence favouring upright posture, it is time to move beyond the soft position of encouraging women to assume whatever posture is comfortable for them. Both the Cochrane review in this area (Gupta *et al.* 2004) and the NICE guidelines (NICE 2007) take up this insipid position in deference to the choice mantra, when the advice, in my view, should be more unequivocal: women are to be encouraged to adopt upright posture, especially in the second stage and for birth. Because bed birth on one's back is still so common in the Western world, I would advocate reframing the information to emphasise the disadvantages of semi-recumbent bed birth:

- decreased fetal oxygenation, lower pH
- increased abnormal fetal heart patterns
- longer second stage
- more likely to have other interventions, e.g. epidural, syntocinon, episiotomy, instrumental births

- less desire to bear down
- smaller outlet diameters
- more severe pain.

These strategies are an unashamed attempt to roll back three or four centuries of birth posture medicalisation that is neither a technological advance on thousands of years of prior, more primitive birth practice, nor an evidence-based alternative to the important principle of attendants fitting around birthing women.

## Context, beds and birth rooms

Of all the clinical apparatus or furniture in the birth room, the bed is the most potent symbol of medicalised birth. In this key area of birth posture, what we do about the bed is a touchstone of our commitment to normal birth and to the principle of the birth attendant as a follower, not a leader. At the end of the 1990s, a manager of an alongside midwifery unit (AMU) reflected on fifteen years of practice as she was about to retire. In particular, she spoke of all those years assisting women to birth in a variety of postures and what she thought of recent trends to limit women's options because of health and safety concerns. She warmed to her theme:

> Over the past 15 years I could count on the fingers of one hand the number of times I may have put my back at risk, even though I have chased women all around the room, mostly low to the floor. There are two reasons for this – firstly I know the principles of good back care and I've found that I could apply them with a bit of lateral thinking to whatever the woman decided to do. It just takes some thinking through. Secondly, I have learnt over the years to let go of my preoccupation with controlling the birth by being down on the floor twisting my neck and spine to see the advancing presenting part. I can use a mirror for that and a baby can slip out on to a soft surface without me having to manipulate everything with my hands. I worry that real reason staff refuse to work on birth centres is less about health and safety concerns and more about unfamiliarity with assisting birth in upright postures. The latter can be easily addressed with training.

It was inspirational to see her challenge the institutional constraints imposed by health and safety and infection control officers, who over the years had tried to limit options in the birth room by condemning carpets, furniture made of wood, birth pools, low mattresses and divans, birth balls and supportive slings. She urged them to shed their generic mindset based on adult surgical/medical wards and contextualise their risk assessments for this entirely different setting of healthy, fit women having normal labours. All over the Western world, similar battles are played out in maternity hospitals.

The ultimate challenge to the ubiquity of the bed comes from home birth where women seldom choose the bed to birth on. Here, where the mirroring of indigenous birth is most manifest, the assumption is not made that the birth room will be the bedroom. Contemporary birth centres have engaged with this truism and many are wonderfully flexible spaces where a woman can construct her own 'nest'. Birth rooms in hospitals can take steps down this path by simply removing beds or positioning them along walls. A number of large obstetric units have taken these steps with some of their birth rooms and the changes have stood the test of time. It's a small step, but a hugely symbolic one.

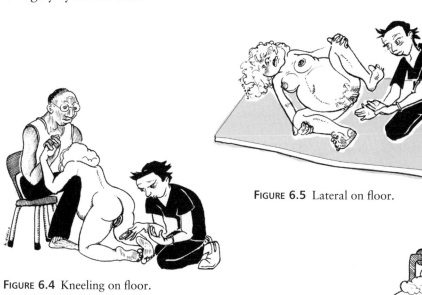

FIGURE 6.5 Lateral on floor.

FIGURE 6.4 Kneeling on floor.

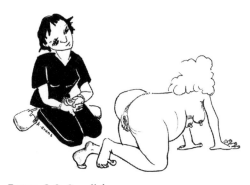

FIGURE 6.6 On all fours.

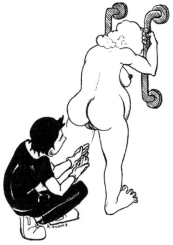

FIGURE 6.7 Standing.

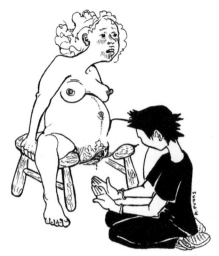

FIGURE 6.8 Birth stool.

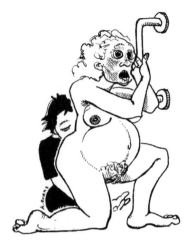

FIGURE 6.9 One leg up.

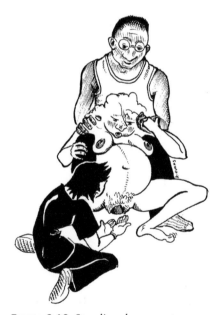

FIGURE 6.10 Standing deep squat.

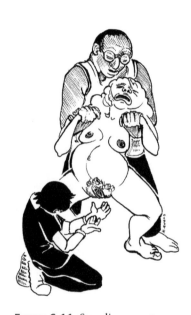

FIGURE 6.11 Standing squat.

## Posture and perineal outcomes

Though there is strong belief among midwives who attend primarily upright births that these positions result in less perineal trauma, until Shorten *et al.*'s (2002) multiple regression analysis no one had examined perineal outcome by different birth posture. Their findings showed lateral posture was associated with the most intact perineums and the fewest episiotomies. All-fours, standing, kneeling and semi-recumbent were all similar in relation to intact perineum. The squatting position, especially for nulliparous women, had the worst outcomes of all positions, though the authors comment that the relatively small sample means these results must be interpreted with caution. Soong and Barnes' (2005) later survey concurred with Shorten's study, except they found that the all-fours position resulted in less suturing.

Shorten and colleagues also examined outcomes by accoucheur and found that births attended by obstetricians were significantly more likely to have episiotomies or sustain perineal trauma. They also commented on extraneous factors known to have a deleterious impact on perineal trauma like increasing birth weight, increasing maternal age, first births and length of the second stage (linked to more episiotomies). More recent research links epidural use and the manner of instructed pushing in the second stage with more trauma (Soong and Barnes 2005, Sampselle *et al.* 2005).

In this context, the amount of room at the pelvic outlet should theoretically have some impact, with upright posture allowing for easier birth of the head and shoulders. It is interesting to note that studies of waterbirth are beginning to show more intact perineums (Geissbuehler *et al.* 2004) and women tend to adopt upright postures in this setting and move more frequently in this medium (Stark *et al.* 2008).

On a tangential but related issue, Downe *et al.*'s (2004) trial of women with epidurals concluded there were more normal vaginal births if women gave birth in lateral postures. Examining the research around epidurals alerts us to the fact that obstetric anaesthetists are looking at ways of harnessing the value of upright posture and movement in labour to reduce the incidence of assisted vaginal births in women with epidurals. The burgeoning research in this area is all predicated on the fact that movement and upright posture are physiologically advantageous to women in labour and, in theory, should facilitate shortened labour and more normal births. Evidence is tentative at this stage but encouraging (Frenea *et al.* 2004, Golara *et al.* 2002).

## Occipito-posterior positions and labour posture

This is an area of much debate among midwives and recent decades have seen a number of theoretical explanations and solutions put forward. Gardberg and Tuppurainen (1994) found the incidence of posterior position was about 10–15 per cent at onset of labour and about 6 per cent at birth. Anecdotally, the number of posterior positions at onset of labour is increasing, with Sutton and Scott (1996) arguing that Western lifestyles are contributing to this. They argue that more sedentary lifestyles, in particular the preponderance of reclining postures that tilt the baby back in the uterus, contribute to this increase. Their solution is more controversial: to encourage forward-tilting postures, sitting upright and side-lying in later pregnancy. Sutton argues from her New Zealand experience that this can virtually eliminate posterior position at the onset of labour, but critics point to the absence of empirical validation to substantiate this claim. As already stated, Hunter *et al.*'s (2007) systematic review was not conclusive as to benefit of the specific knee/chest position in later pregnancy.

While a trial of Sutton's package of care is needed, I support her dissemination of her approach at workshops where she argues cogently from physiology and anatomy in support of her principles for optimal fetal positioning. Her arguments simply have strong intuitive appeal and resonance with what we know of fetal alignment and descent of the presenting part through the curve of Carus (*Midirs* 2004).

More recently, the role of aquanatal exercises in facilitating occipito-anterior position at the beginning of labour has been raised by Baines (2010). Her audit of women passing through her aquanatal classes over a two-year period indicates an extremely low incidence of posterior position at birth, especially in nulliparous women. We know that rates of persistent posterior position in this group are increased by epidural use (Lieberman *et al.* 2005) and it is no surprise that Baines' cohort of women went on to use hydrotherapy during labour with many having waterbirths, thus avoiding epidurals.

Simkin and Ancheta (2011), in their important book on labour progress, suggest a number of strategies to address persistent posterior position during labour and the majority are positional manoeuvres. The lunge (creating disequilibrium between the hips through the use of steps) and the hip squeeze are two. Shallow (2003) has written of applications for this condition using a birth ball. Finally, Frye (2004) addresses it in her comprehensive home birth manual, describing the technique of creating a false pelvic floor during vaginal examination to help rotate the fetal head. I will return to this topic in the chapter on the second stage of labour (Chapter 8).

## Upright posture and assisted vaginal birth

I have encountered four instances over the past three years of women having ventouse or lift-out forceps birth in an upright posture. The postures were all-fours, standing (leaning over a bed) and a supported squat.

In each case, the obstetricians and midwives flexed to accommodate the women's desire to birth upright. On one occasion, after traction to bring the head down to the perineum, the ventouse cap was released so the woman could birth spontaneously. There was a wonderful narrative in the *Midirs Digest* recently that gave the perspectives of all those present at one of these births (Byrom, Fardella *et al.* 2010). It is inspirational to read. For obstetricians, they have to think through the direction of traction which is reversed from the conventional lithotomy pose. It does not make the procedure more technical or complex but does require them to move out of the comfort zone of convention. One recent association appearing more often in the literature that supports this more flexible approach is that between lithotomy position and anal sphincter tear (Dudding *et al.* 2008).

## Birth position and educational initiatives

Exposure to antenatal education packages has traditionally been a poor predictor of a reduction in birth intervention rates (Nolan 2005). However, like Baines' aquanatal package, current programmes in many services in the UK are explicitly premised on an active birth philosophy and there is some evidence that these are beginning to make a difference to women's choices around birth posture. Foster's (2005) BirthTalk programme consisted of a two-hour education session for women and their birth companions, facilitated by a midwife, and had the following characteristics:

- held in a birth suite room within the hospital when women were thirty-four weeks' gestation;
- ice-breaker exercises;
- interactive teaching with doll and pelvis on mechanism of labour, 'powers, passages, passenger' explored, supported by video;
- practising of labour postures with partner support;
- small-group work on expectations and birth plan;
- size limited to five couples.

Her evaluation showed a remarkable 30 per cent increase in upright posture for birth and 50 per cent reduction in epidurals compared with a similar group of women who did not access the programme.

Keys to the success of this programme probably lie in exposing women to posture possibilities in late pregnancy in an environment they are likely to be labouring in. Practising positions and troubleshooting queries in a small group would have also contributed. It is clearly far superior to having this conversation with women already labouring as many midwives have to do in the current system.

The other target for education is midwives themselves. Many midwives access skills-based workshops in this area, but they are commonly those already convinced of their value. In the late 1990s, I was involved in a collaborative audit project that aimed at improving midwives' care in areas where strong evidence existed. We addressed skills for supporting upright birth posture by running Robertson's Active Birth workshops (Robertson 1997). Midwives from a cross-section of experiences and philosophies attended, and when we re-measured practice after a month of educational initiatives, the number of women adopting an upright posture for birth had risen by 12 per cent, a modest but encouraging result (Walsh *et al.* 1999).

## Conclusion

Being free to move and change posture is of paramount importance for normal labour and birth physiology. We know this from myriad sources, but probably the most profound is that intuitive reservoir of embodied knowledge that women have expressed in childbirth for millennia. Across cultures and across epochs, the restlessness of labour manifested and it is only in the modern era that this ancient wisdom has been challenged. There is a breathtaking arrogance about this challenge that saw the folly of birth on one's back on a bed exported to the developing world, precisely where birth practices in this area remained connected to the ancient wisdom. In recent years, Western birth practices have sought an evidence route out of this arrogance by testing the efficacy of mobility and upright posture. And now we know what others knew all along.

In correcting the wrongs of decades of managed birth, forthright measures are required. Removing beds from normal birth rooms would be a potent marker of intent but we also need to re-educate the childbirth professionals so that they are facilitators of physiology, not manipulators of it, and so that they create birth environments that encourage uninhibited expression of all the senses, not professional spaces on loan to women who have little control over its boundaries. There is a synergism that needs to happen here around physiological behaviours within a woman's safe birth space. Only then will labouring women's intuitive movement and posture find full freedom.

## Practice recommendations

- Women need to be informed of advantages of upright postures and disadvantages of recumbent postures.
- Midwives should fit around women, not the other way round.
- Midwives need to gain competence and confidence in assisting women with upright postures.
- Props should be provided that facilitate upright postures.
- Positions need practice antenatally, preferably in the birth room that is likely to be used.
- Antenatal active birth classes should be available for women.

- Aquanatal exercise provision should be an option for women.
- Conventional beds should be removed from normal birth rooms.
- Women should be informed that EFM, IVs and epidurals affect mobility.
- If labour is prolonged, mobility/postural change could be of benefit.
- Mobility and upright postures should be encouraged with modern epidurals.

**Questions for reflection**

How could you 'make over' birth rooms to facilitate posture/position flexibility?

How could you address the removal of conventional beds for birth rooms?

How could you apply the principle of attendants fitting around women regarding position/posture?

How can midwifery skills assist the dissemination of upright postures?

Is there a need for you to review antenatal classes to address active birth education and the opportunity to simulate postures in the likely birth room?

# Chapter 7 **Pain and labour**

- Pain, birthing and context
- Models of labour pain
- Psychological methods
- Physical therapies
- Sensory methods
- Complementary therapies
- Spiritual rituals
- Technologies and drugs
- Conclusion
- Practice recommendations
- Questions for reflection

I was shocked about how painful it was … right at the end when I was pushing, I just wanted them to cut me open. I'd just had enough. The pain was unbelievable, I really didn't think it was going to hurt like that … like a knife being pushed up your backside…. But the moment he come out it was just the most unbelievable experience. And you just keep reliving it for days. The pain was like forgotten then. Brilliant, an amazing experience, nothing touches it … all of a sudden you just come alive.

(Liz, first baby in a birth centre)

This poignant quotation about a woman's experience of birth in a birth centre captures the paradox inherent in childbirth pain – the agony and the ecstasy. It leads us into the heart of the conundrum regarding pain and the contemporary experience of childbirth, at least in the Western world. Though pain is intrinsic to labour, in most other contexts of our lives it is seen as negative and treatable by a variety of pharmacological agents. A whole sub-specialism of anaesthetics has evolved in maternity care to devise increasingly sophisticated and technological solutions to labour pain. From this perspective, the development is part of a medicalisation of childbirth that has been ongoing over the past 200 years or so.

The availability of epidural anaesthesia, arguably the most successful of these technological advances, and its increasing uptake, poses a question that would have been unthinkable 200 years ago – how can women do labour without one? With rates for primigravid women at 70 per cent in some units, it does seem a reasonable question to ask and yet, for the midwife, the question highlights how far the maternity services and society's expectations have shifted from an anthropological understanding of childbirth towards the biomedical paradigm. Yet, research has consistently shown that dissatisfaction with birth is seldom related to the intensity of pain (Hodnett 2002). In fact, a body of research shows the opposite – that coping with labour pain is associated with feelings of self-esteem (Callister et al. 2003, Niven and Murphy-Black 2000) and self-growth (Aldrich and Eccleston 2000).

In this chapter I will revisit the debate around pain and labour raised in the first edition, during the course of which I will, once again, draw on Leap and Anderson's (2008) seminal writing on models of labour pain. I will then examine the evidence base of a whole spectrum of supportive measures and interventions, from psychological methods to physical therapies, from sensory aids to complementary therapies and from birth environment issues to pharmacological agents.

## Pain, birthing and context

Mander (2001) argues powerfully that RCTs that examined doula-style care offering one-to-one support in labour were effectively a sop to ameliorate the

iatrogenic effects of medicalised birth. In other words, doula care was introduced to humanise the medicalised face of modern intrapartum provision.
Though these studies concluded that one-to-one support reduced the need
for pharmacological analgesia, such findings are not surprising given the
abysmal birthing conditions women laboured in. Her point is that there is a
more fundamental problem here to do with inappropriate medicalisation of
birth and a grossly dysfunctional organisational birthing culture. A focus on
technology, a focus on task and record-keeping, an institutionalised and bureaucratic milieu, absence of privacy and of known birth companions, rigid
policies and protocols conspire to make large hospital maternity units toxic
for normal birth.

Disappointingly, thirty years on from these original doula studies, many of
the same conditions still exist, especially around fragmented models of care
and the inability to provide one-to-one labour care. When I spoke out about
rising epidural rates in low-risk women in 2009 (*Observer* 2009), I wanted
to highlight this failing in many UK labour wards, despite decades of
research stating that continuous support in labour is the most powerful intervention of all. We have to address the birthing culture if we are ever going to
challenge the increasing reliance on pain-relieving drugs in labour.

It is necessary to continually restate that large consultant units are inevitably hostile places for normal birth and that small midwifery-led birth
centres and the increasing availability of home birth must expand if we are
to fundamentally shift the biomedical paradigm towards a social model of
care. Downsizing has the advantage of personalising a service. There is more
time to individualise care and more time to build relationships, both key
dimensions of labour care. Mander (2001), in her review of labour support
studies, found many instances where actual one-on-one time between midwives and women was in single-figure percentages. The rest of the time they
were serving the institution's needs in a variety of tasks from record-keeping,
to giving reports, to attending to birth technologies like electronic fetal monitoring, to running errands for other staff. A midwife's continuous support
with a woman was always what was compromised whenever any other task
arose, like attending to medical staff requests. She simply left the women and
prioritised the doctor's needs. Mander also noted that a number of hospital-
based, shift-working midwives chose to spend time socialising with other
staff outside the room rather than with the woman she was allocated to.
Caseload midwifery models reveal a different dynamic of midwives accompanying a woman into the delivery rooms from home and then remaining
with her for the majority of the time (Walsh 1999).

Changing the institutional setting and even altering the ways midwives
work still does not deal with the paradigm shift required from viewing birth

as primarily a medical event to understanding it as a 'rite-of-passage' transition – the former viewing pain as an optional extra that one can choose to dispense with and the latter embracing it as integral to the physiology of childbirth and intrinsic to psychological growth. To capture the anthropological perspective, I reproduce Anderson's poetic reflection on her experiences of physiological birth:

> If you are privileged enough to have witnessed a woman giving birth unaided in a place she has chosen, what will you have seen? You will first be in awe of her strength. Her thighs stand strong and mighty like those of a warrior as she stands, sways and squats to find the best position to ease her baby out. Then you will hear the deep primal cries she makes as she does her work, sounds that come not from her throat but from her belly as she grunts and moans with her exertion: sounds seldom heard except in the most uninhibited of love-making. Maybe you will notice the glistening river of mucous tinged with blood and waters that run down her thighs unheeded: she is beyond noticing such things, moved as she has done into another plane of existence. And then finally you will be struck by her beauty: her face softened with the flow of oxytocin, her eyes wide and shining, her pupils dark, deep and open. And you will think – for how could you not – what a phenomenal creature is a woman. But you will only have seen this astonishing sight if you understand that if you disturb her in her work, she will be thrown off course. Like a zoologist, you must first learn how to behave; how to sit quietly and patiently, almost invisible, breathing with her, not disturbing her mighty internal rhythm. And you will see that the pain of her labours seldom overwhelms her. Nature would not have organised labour to be intolerable.
>
> (Leap and Anderson 2008, p. 34)

Adopting this lens to labour will change the intrinsic orientation of both women and midwives. To flesh out ideas around this alternative lens, Leap and Anderson's (2008) juxtaposing of 'pain relief' and 'working with pain' models is very helpful. They suggest the majority of maternity services adopt a 'pain relief' approach to labour pain. Table 7.1 contrasts the ideas in each.

## Models of labour pain

More recently, Leap has summarised her understanding of this approach for the NCT in the UK (Leap 2010). The subtleties of language are embedded in the managed birth culture and it will continue to be a struggle to

TABLE 7.1

| Pain-relief approach | Working with pain approach |
|---|---|
| • Language suggestive of pain as a problem | • Language suggestive of pain as normative |
| • Paternalistic, 'we can protect you from unnecessary stress' | • Egalitarian empowerment, 'we are alongside you' |
| • Techno/rationalism age, pain is preventable/treatable | • Labour pain timeless component of 'rite-of-passage' transitions |
| • Neutral impact of environment | • Seminal impact of environment |
| • Clinical expertise of professional carers | • Supportive role of birth companions |
| • Special session/focus in antenatal education | • Woven throughout labour preparation sessions |
| • 'Menu approach' to options for coping with pain | • Supportive strategies for journey of labour |
| • Pain as a 'management issue' for assembly-line birth | • Pain as one dimension of labour care in one-to-one, small-scale birth settings |
| • Contributes to trend of rising epidural rates | • Contributes to trend to less pharmacological analgesia |
| • Risks of pharmacological agents outweighed by benefits | • 'Cascade of intervention' dynamic |
| • First birth special case for 'menu approach' | • First birth optimal opportunity for 'working with pain' |
| • Informed choice means all options must be presented | • Informed choice within context of birthing plan and philosophy |

unmask it in hospital birth, where the recording of the birth event in maternal notes remains dominated by biomedical language. We need to find new ways of using words so that they cease grounding us in a clinical mindset. Roberts *et al.* (2010) make a start with their 'coping with labour algorithm', which is a tool midwives use in labour. They deliberately use the word 'labour' rather than 'pain', and coping mechanisms embrace the environment, the psychosocial/emotional and the physiology of labour, with the latter divided into non-pharmacological interventions and pharmacological interventions.

A 'working with pain' approach helps us recognise that there are a number of rationales for labour pain. It alerts women to the start of labour, prompting them to seek a safe place for birth as all mammals do and, uniquely for humans, appropriate companions. It plays a crucial role in the neuro-hormonal cascade of labour, detailed in Chapter 4, which progresses the labour at the appropriate rate for the individual woman. Part of this mechanism is the endorphin effect of endogenous opiates (McLean *et al.* 1994) which the midwife needs to be able to recognise in physiological labour. These are primarily manifested by movement, ecstatic experiences and an altered state of consciousness (Ribeiro *et al.* 2005). Labour pain gives clues to the birth attendant as to the rhythms of labour, foreshadowing the movement from early labour to active labour and the later transition prior to the second stage. Its varying intensity may hint at latent phases of rest and finally its severity to possible pathology. The ability to discern physiological from pathological pain is an important skill for the midwife to develop and arguably is best accrued by routine exposure to non-medicated, normal labour.

Pain has significant psychosocial ramifications. Its impact and the woman's successful journey through it to birth marks the occasion out as life-changing, even transformational, and with the potential for personal growth. The enormity of this achievement may be qualitatively different from anaesthetised labour or an elective caesarean section. One has only to witness the intensity of emotions expressed at physiological labour and birth to recognise this. Joy is one of the most obvious, and yet it is rarely mentioned in professional texts on childbirth. Relief and triumph can be present in equal measure. These emotions are often shared by the midwife who has witnessed first hand over many hours the courage, vulnerability and strength of women. In some cultures, the achievement of physiological birth is highlighted through spiritual rituals that give meaning to the pain as redemptive and preparatory for motherhood. Thomson and Downe's (2010) research demonstrated this powerfully in their study of positive birth experiences following previous traumatic births. A woman used the phrase 'changing the future to change the past' when reflecting on the impact of her positive birth experience. Odent (2001) and others have written of the reciprocal hormonal surges in mothers and babies at birth, noting the high level of endorphins in both which may facilitate mutual 'addiction' to each other. All of these factors probably facilitate early bonding with babies in the hours following birth.

Internalising the 'working with pain' approach is an important step for midwives steeped in the 'pain relief' modality. It assists them in being with labouring women in pain while remaining comfortable with their own response. As a student midwife commented, reflecting on her disproportionate exposure to medicalised birth: 'I am concerned that firstly I will not learn to recognise the normal manifestation and parameters of physiological labour pain and secondly that it will traumatise me to witness it.'

This kind of pain is different from the artificial pain of an induced or augmented labour. Taylor's (1990) poem captures eloquently the syntocinon effect:

The electric pump clicks, drip fed through the meter
by clear plastic tubes and a needle jammed into my vein
This is not my body's pain.
It does not rise like breath or the fierce arched rainbows
I have imagined.
From a burning bush it spreads like forest fire
with me in front of it, running.

To cope with this chemically enhanced pain, epidural anaesthesia is probably appropriate.

I have mentioned already that the physical environment and the style of care play a key part in how women respond to labour pain. Research on home birth (Janssen *et al.* 2009), free-standing birth centres (Walsh and Downe 2004) and integrated birth centres (Hodnett *et al.* 2010) all conclude that less pharmacological analgesia is used in these settings. Research into midwifery-led models of care comes to the same conclusion (Hatem *et al.* 2008) and Hodnett *et al.*'s (2009) review of continuous support in labour is also consistent in its findings of less analgesia. Leap *et al.* (2010) has demonstrated the importance of relational continuity within the caseload midwifery model in reducing dramatically the need for any labour analgesia. More interesting research on labour support explored the effect of untrained female companions, linking their effectiveness to 'tending and befriending' behaviours, also mentioned in Chapter 3 (Rosen 2004). I am becoming increasingly convinced that the choice of appropriate birth companions is fundamental for the positive experience of physiological labour and that may mean that the male partner is not the best choice for this role unless they have had training.

---

**Box 7.1** Helpful strategies for enhancing this role should include:

- belief in the value of normal labour and birth;
- belief that women can 'do it';
- previous exposure to normal labour and birth as an observer/assistant or as a mother;
- prior relationship established with the woman;
- awareness of the woman's birth plan;
- planned strategies of support.

---

With these considerations addressed, all of what I now go on to explore are given optimal conditions to work.

Some final thoughts before exploring the evidence base of various support strategies: women vary enormously in their perception of pain and there are many factors that impinge on this perception, among them the cultural diversity highlighted eloquently by Callister *et al.* (2003) in their interviews of women from four different continents. The midwife who knows the woman in her care is clearly at an enormous advantage here, though developing instant rapport-building skills is learned early on in one's midwifery career. Second, as already mentioned, there is not a direct relationship between decreasing pain and increasing satisfaction. The paradox of childbirth means both can co-exist and be rated highly.

## Psychological methods

Facilitating a woman's ability to relax has been a cornerstone of antenatal education for several decades. There is a lack of research evidence in support of relaxation in its many guises and techniques, but common sense and intuition tells us that it is a worthwhile strategy. It can reduce anxiety, body tension and the excess secretion of stress hormones that may render a labour dysfunctional. Dick-Read (1957) is credited with systematising an approach (psychoprophylaxis) built around relaxation techniques and providing education as to what to expect. He had a clear rationale for this to do with interrupting the fear–pain–more fear–more pain cycle, and his approach became very popular in the USA in the 1930s before being exported to the UK. The Active Birth Movement refined his approach in the 1970s and 1980s in the UK, adding training on birth posture and breathing techniques (Balaskas 1990).

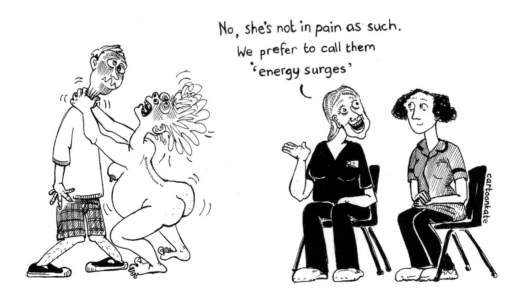

Chapter 2 explored the evidence base of antenatal education broadly, concluding that tentative evidence is beginning to emerge supporting its effectiveness in reducing the use of pain-relieving drugs in labour, but this cannot be linked solely to relaxation techniques. In recent years, variants of the technique, especially those related to hypnosis, have begun to emerge with a more substantial traditional evidence base. Cyna and colleagues (2004) systematically reviewed trials of hypnosis and found that they did reduce the need for analgesia, including epidurals and narcotics, in individual studies. Many women rated their pain as being less severe. The authors suggest that new forms of hypnosis that emphasise self-inducing the trance state may enhance women's sense of control. Accompanying the research has been an explosion in web resources on hypno-birthing (www.gentlebirth.org/archives/hypnosis.html), together with a renewed interest by midwives in these techniques (Mottershead 2006). Reading the literature around hypno-birthing, one is struck by an underlying philosophy that emphasises women's empowerment and enhancing labour physiology.

Related to relaxation techniques and hypnosis is the use of imagery and neuro-linguistic programming (NLP) to orient women to approaching labour optimistically and to reframe fears and anxieties positively (Spencer 2005, Camm 2006). There is no research on these approaches as yet, but the resonance with Green et al.'s (1998) findings that expectations of birth shape actual experiences is noteworthy.

Mack (2000) encourages midwives and women to consider the Alexander Technique to facilitate relaxation during labour. An approach specifically designed for professional musicians and vocalists, it combines breathing techniques with an awareness of body posture to induce calm prior to performance. More information is available from www.alexandertechnique.com.

It is worth mentioning here the potential value of music in augmenting relaxation and contributing to a calming ambience. Cepeda et al.'s (2006) systematic review of music for pain relief in any condition showed it reduced pain intensity and the need for opioids. Research has also demonstrated the anxiolytic effect of music (Spintge 1989) and Browning's (2000) small study, specific to labour care, showed women found it a helpful strategy for coping with labour pain and stress. A later trial (Browning 2001) revealed that women were more relaxed and perceived greater control in the music therapy group. Rhythmical movement during labour is a common occurrence and music is likely to facilitate this, though it is an area where individual taste will vary.

## Physical therapies

The use of supportive touch in labour is extremely common and is both symbolic as a conduit of connection between labour companions and the woman and therapeutic as an empathic physical response to a body in pain. There is a certain instinctiveness to cradling or massaging the injured part. At this level, physical touch simply 'works' if desired by the woman and has no need of a traditional evidence base. It is well to remind ourselves of this from time to time and to act both instinctively and intuitively in labour care, always cognisant of the woman's response.

Of course, physical practices of massage have spawned a variety of techniques, each claiming particular benefits, and it is therefore important to examine the evidence we have to date. Khoda Karami et al.'s (2007) study showed that massaging the back and limbs of women in labour significantly lowered pain levels, reduced the need for pain relief and reduced labour length. Yildirim and Sahin (2004) also found that massage reduced pain levels in every phase of labour. Chang et al. (2002) randomised women to a package of massage that included abdominal effleurage, sacral pressure and shoulder/back kneading. This group experienced significantly less pain reactions and anxiety than the control group for the latent, active and transitional phases of labour. The authors also commented on the benefit to labour carers who were able to contribute in positive way to supporting their partners. Field et al.'s (1997) small trial showed remarkable effects in the massage group, including decreased depressed mood, anxiety and pain, less agitated activity, shorter labours, shorter hospital stay and less postnatal depression. However, the small sample size merits the study being repeated with larger numbers.

Movement and posture change are other behaviours in labour that beg the question of why they should be considered 'interventions' that require evaluation at all. Gould (2000) stated what observers of normal labour have known, probably for millennia, that movement is intrinsic to its presentation and that what really needs evaluating is the intervention of immobilisation on a bed. There may be no better example of the perverse logic and counterintuitive thrust of medically managed birth than the series of trials over the last thirty years that have examined mobility and positional change in labour. These studies tested the experimental intervention of freedom to move and upright posture compared with standard, conventional care of labouring on a bed on your back! It will come as no surprise that these studies concluded that mobility and upright posture reduced the need for pharmacological analgesia and increased childbirth satisfaction (Simkin and O'Hara 2002). This has been reinforced by Lawrence et al.'s (2009) systematic review of mobility in the first stage of labour, which clearly demonstrated a lowering of epidural rates and a shortening of labour. Additionally, Spiby *et al.* (2003) concluded that position impacts on a woman's sense of control. In reference specifically to women with occipito-posterior positions during labour, Stremler and colleagues (2005) found that the knee/chest position, adopted for thirty minutes during labour, significantly reduced persistent back pain, and I covered this topic in the chapter on labour and birth postures.

There is now evidence of the value of antenatal yoga for increasing feelings of comfort and reducing pain intensity in labour (Chuntharapat *et al.* 2008). In addition, the women studied had shorter labours. Less common, but with similar potential for benefit, is the exploration of dance as a mode of physical expression during labour. There are glimpses of synergetic effects here, as music would commonly accompany dance.

## Sensory methods

If there is one area where the evidence base has moved ahead apace in the last five years it is hydrotherapy. Cluett *et al.*'s (2004) RCT was a landmark publication which challenged the orthodoxy that slow labour would only respond to syntocinon augmentation, with the inevitable rise in the uptake of epidural anaesthesia. They showed that slow labours responded better to water immersion than to syntocinon and that epidural rate reduced as a consequence. In an observational study of over 12,000 births, Eberhard *et al.* (2005) concluded that more women who used water immersion had no analgesia during labour than women who laboured on beds. The latter group had more epidurals in late labour. Water immersion reduced mean labour pain scores in Da Silva *et al.*'s trial (2009). Earlier, Hall and Holloway (1998) had shown that women who laboured in water had a high sense of control, and again we see the synergetic effects of related factors coming together.

Aromatherapy is another sensory-style intervention for labour care that benefits from a large study (Burns *et al.* 2000). Her study of 9000 women in Oxford showed a reduction in opioid use, with a majority of women stating it was helpful. Burns *et al.* (2007) undertook a pilot RCT in Italy and found lower pain scores in those who experienced water immersion. Similar conclusions were reached by Mousely (2005) after an audit of the aromatherapy service at her hospital. She also found that staff were enthusiastic about the service. Aromatherapy is commonly combined with hydrotherapy and/or massage, both of which may augment its effects.

Gaskin, Kitzinger and latterly Buckley have argued over recent decades for a more thorough examination of the place of sexual expression in labour care, convincingly elucidating their complementary physiology and anatomy. Buckley (2010), in particular, in her comprehensive coverage of sexual and birth hormones, remind us of the endorphin-like effects of clitoral stimulation and orgasm, posing the important question of why these practices are rarely observed or encouraged in birth rooms. The only research reported to date is Gaskin's (2002) survey of the incidence of orgasm in normal labour, where 20 per cent of women described orgasm-like experiences. It seems a denial of potential benefit that sexual behaviours are uncommon in Western birth, which undoubtedly has much to do with environmental and cultural inhibitions and taboos. These need to be addressed if a truly holistic appreciation of labour and birth is to be embraced.

## Complementary therapies

I now want to examine, in no particular order, the evidence base of common complementary therapies that are practised during labour. These are inevitably selective as there are myriad therapies available.

The trials on acupuncture are summarised in Smith *et al.* (2006) and show a decrease in pharmacological analgesia, including epidural. A more recent RCT (Borup *et al.* 2009) confirmed these findings. In the studies, obstetric anaesthetists only used acupuncture, but many midwives have trained in its use and practise regularly. In some Swedish maternity units, over 70 per cent of midwives have undertaken the training and, in the UK, Denny (1999) has published an audit of her practice. Yelland's text *Acupuncture in Midwifery* (2005) remains one of the best resources on the market for midwives with an interest in this area.

It is important to make the general point that recognised accreditation now exists for many complementary therapies, and there are numerous examples of local policies and procedures defining their scope of practice. This should encourage midwives who have an interest in particular practices to seek qualification. In the past this has been a tortuous route of overcoming resistance and obstacles to eventually gaining permission to practise. However, in most cases now it should not be necessary to 'reinvent the wheel', as almost certainly other maternity units have practitioners who have done this already. Professional midwifery bodies in each country probably have a database of these midwives. Mitchell and Williams (2006) have written eloquently about the challenge to maternity services of incorporating complementary therapies into their package of provision.

The related therapy of acupressure or shiatsu has had two RCTs published that found that acupressure reduced labour pain scores and the length of labour (Kyeong *et al.* 2004, Hjelmstedt *et al.* 2010). There was also a trend to lower uptake of analgesia. In a very specific modification of shiatsu, Waters and Raisler (2003) demonstrated pain reduction when massaging the hand using an ice bag placed on the large intestine meridian point near the thumb. Yates (2003) has written extensively about shiatsu's application to maternity care, stressing its psychological benefits of reducing anxiety and increasing energy levels. Western paradigms of pain control mechanisms struggle to accept these ancient Chinese medicine practices which come with an alternative physiology. Variations on the 'gate control' mechanism and natural endorphin release have been used to explain their effects.

Finally, reflexology fits within this group of therapies, using the same ancient Chinese physiology of meridian lines or zones representing energy flows throughout the body and the importance of keeping these in balance. Reflexology specifically links reflex zones on the feet and toes to organ systems in the body, so that applying certain 'grip' sequences will stimulate the body to self-heal organ dysfunction (Tiran and Mack 2000). Two studies of uncertain robustness suggest that the need for analgesia and labour length is reduced in women having reflexology in labour (Liisberg 1989, Motha and McGrath 1993).

Homeopathy, based on the principle that 'like cures like' and emphasising the body's self-healing properties, has a long history of medicinal use in the UK. The research base for labour care is paltry, with only one study suggesting that caulophyllum reduced the duration of labour (Eid *et al.* 1993). Both Stockton (2003) and Cummings and Tiran (2000) have written about its use in maternity care, with the latter authors suggesting that chamomilla reduced irritability and sensitivity to pain. Practitioners of homeopathy stress, as do many complementary therapists, the importance of a holistic approach, and this is certainly an attitude that traditional Western medicine could learn from.

Herbalism has the inherent appeal of using naturally occurring organic plants and has an ancient history, representing some of the earliest treatments of primitive medicine. Despite this, there is almost a total absence of any conventional evidence base. The notable exception was Calvert's (2005) small RCT of the use of ginger oil to shorten labour, suggesting an effect in the second stage of labour. One could argue that thousands of years of use for specific conditions is more than an adequate evidence substitute for the modern-day RCT, which has been with us for less than fifty years. It is in this spirit that I summarise Stapleton and Tiran's (2000) recommendations of herbal remedies for labour. They suggest ginger root, raspberry leaf tea, rosemary or ginseng to help restore energy during long labours and may therefore impact on analgesic use. These come in a variety of preparations.

A final point that is worth mentioning in relation to complementary therapies is their general focus on enhancing health and preventing illness, as opposed to conventional medicine's orientation to curing disease and ameliorating symptoms. This resonates with physiological childbirth as a state of health and a powerful expression of well-being, not illness or potential pathology.

## Spiritual rituals

The consideration of the potential place of spirituality in the labour experience is of only secondary consideration in Western-style birth. In indigenous cultures and in settings where birth operates more within a social model, the spiritual marking of birth is commonplace (Kitzinger 2000, Hall 2001). I raise it in the context of pain because the small amount of literature we do have addressing the topic engages centrally with pain and its meaning. Thomas (2001) reflects on her Roman Catholic faith to interpret labour pain as cleansing and redemptive, in parallel to the suffering of Jesus. This is tricky territory because the Church was criticised during the nineteenth century for opposing the use of chloroform during birth because it violated the Old Testament maxim that childbirth would be accompanied by travail. In Kitzinger's travel through traditional birthing cultures, she observed the rich and ancient spiritual beliefs around goddesses and the sacredness of childbirth. These had incredible power to sanctify the woman in the wondrous creative act of childbirth.

With a renewal of interest in spirituality, though not necessarily in organised religion, opportunities to explore childbirth from this perspective should be examined. These may assist in rehabilitating the sense of the sacred in birth, diminished by medicalisation over recent decades. Rossiter-Thornton's (2002) prayer wheel is a tool that can open up discussion of spirituality without invoking the perspectives of specific world faiths. It is generic in raising dimensions of spirituality rooted in an individual's experience that may stimulate meaning-making around the labour event.

## Technologies and drugs

Transcutaneous Electrical Nerve Stimulation (TENS) has been used in labour for a few decades now. Carroll *et al.*'s (1997) systematic review was pessimistic regarding the value of TENS as a pain-relieving agent, concluding only weak positive effects. (There was some evidence of secondary analgesic sparing and that women expressed a preference to use it for future labours.) Their summary that 'RCTs provide no compelling evidence for TENS having any analgesic effect during labour' illustrates the susceptibility of trials to subjective interpretation. The method, premised on objectivity and the elimination of bias, fails to take seriously the inevitable reflexive posture of authors influencing trial interpretation. Here, maternal preference is deemed a tertiary outcome and undervalued in the summation of the study.

Mander (2011), a midwife, in contrast emphasises the popularity of TENS with women, which offsets to some extent the methodological weaknesses in many of the studies and also picks up on the evidence suggesting it has a positive effect on breastfeeding (Rajan 1994).

One unusual injection that has been shown to be effective in reducing back pain in labour is tiny increments of sterile water. Amounts of 0.5 ml are injected cutaneously into the lower back. Two systematic reviews in recent years have concluded they provide powerful analgesic relief, of the order of 60 per cent reduction in pain (Martensson and Wallin 2008, Fogarty 2008). The duration of effect is approximately two hours.

The ubiquity of entonox or the combination of nitrous oxide and oxygen (in varying concentrations) in birth rooms tells us something of its popularity with midwives. Whether this translated to effectiveness remained unanswered, at least from the perspective of research studies, until Rosen's (2002) systematic review. His rather muted endorsement was that it appears to provide effective analgesia. Again this must be weighed against extremely high ratings of satisfaction (around 85 per cent). This may be due to self-administration and the ability to regulate intake. Some have suggested it works powerfully as a distracting agent, engaging kinaesthetic and, to a lesser extent, auditory faculties. Some critics (Robertson 1997) take the view that women are inhaling a drug with unknown side-effects while others point to its rapid absorption and excretion as reassuring. An exploratory epidemiological study by Jacobson *et al.* (1988) hypothesised a link in later life to amphetamine addiction in babies exposed to entonox but this remains speculative. There may be a sense that its ready availability in a birthing culture focused on the 'pain relief' paradigm and where there are limited pharmacological alternatives reinforces its popularity with both childbirth attendants and women in the absence of convincing evidence.

Opioid use in labour was probably waning in the Western world with the widespread uptake of epidural anaesthesia until fentanyl's incorporation into the epidural cocktail. Over the years narcotics like pethidine and diamorphine and their derivatives have been extensively researched, primarily by anaesthetists. The current Cochrane review of these preparations via the intramuscular route concludes that there is not enough evidence to evaluate comparative efficacy and safety (Ullman *et al.* 2010). Pethidine was used as the control in most studies and seems to remain the most common opiate, though regional and national variations exist with the use of diamorphine and morphine compared with pethidine. Ullman *et al.*'s review indicates that pethidine may cause more nausea, vomiting and drowsiness. On the whole, opiates are a poor analgesic and probably have more profound anaesthetic effects (McInnes *et al.* 2004). Their side-effects are significant:

Fetal effects:

- respiratory depression
- possible opiate addiction in adult life (Jacobson *et al.* 1990)
- diminishes breast-seeking and breastfeeding behaviours (Ransjo-Arvidson *et al.* 2001).

Maternal effects:

- fentanyl reduces likelihood of breastfeeding (Jordan *et al.* 2005)
- euphoria and dysphoria
- nausea/vomiting, slow gastric emptying
- drowsiness/amnesia (Ullman *et al.* 2010)
- longer first and second stage of labour (Mander 2011).

Narcotics continue to be widely available in maternity hospitals. Pethidine in particular is cheap and in many places can be prescribed by midwives, which contributes to its continued popularity. Commonly given in combination with an antiemetic, it remains a largely unsatisfactory analgesic. Heelbeck (1999) suggested that giving smaller increments frequently into the deltoid muscle would accelerate its systemic uptake and diminish its peak-and-trough effects, but this practice is not common.

Intravenous remifentanil is beginning to be researched and used more in some maternity hospitals, largely as an alternative to epidurals. Early systematic reviews indicate that it is of moderate effectiveness and carries the same side-effects as other opioids, in particular oxygen saturation levels need monitoring in the mother (Hinova and Fernando 2009).

Intramuscular narcotics would always struggle to compete with regional epidural anaesthesia once the latter became increasingly available, and that appears to remain the case. This is because of the relative effectiveness of the epidural as a pain-relieving agent compared with the opiates. I will examine its evidence base next.

Anim-Somuah *et al.*'s (2006) Cochrane review rather surprisingly was only able to examine one study comparing the effectiveness of epidural with non-epidural methods of pain relief, though twenty-one studies were identified by the review. This showed that the epidural offered better pain relief. The remainder of the review discusses the possible complications of epidurals and this struck me as an accurate reflection of the context for appraising epidurals. The established associations are:

- need for more oxytocin
- increased length of the second stage of labour
- increase in instrumental birth
- hypotension
- pyrexia.

In addition there are two other associations, not mentioned in the review but established in other literature: an increased incidence of dystocia in low-risk nulliparous women (Kjaergaard *et al.* 2008) and an increased incidence of posterior position at birth after controlling for confounders (Lieberman *et al.* 2005). Finally, there are a number of more tentative associations: increase in urinary stress incontinence (Rortveit, Kjersti *et al.* 2003), anal sphincter tears in nulliparous women (Donnelly *et al.* 1998), fetal tachycardia (Lieberman and O'Donoghue 2002) and reduced breastfeeding rates on discharge (Wiklund *et al.* 2009).

Left out of all these papers was any engagement with a number of other effects that epidurals have on the woman that midwives are confronted with every day on busy labour wards. These include:

- the passivity and 'patient' status that the receiving of an epidural seems to usher in;
- the restrictions on mobility and the tethering to the bed;
- the negating of second-stage physiology and all the frustration inherent in 'coaching' second-stage behaviours;
- the medicalisation of bladder care;
- the imperative to electronically monitor the fetal heart;
- the increasing amount of time spent in technical measurement, observation and record keeping;
- the profound medicalisation of labour and birth that follows from all of the above.

Given these associations and the context of looking after women with epidurals, most midwives consider that epidurals render the labour non-physiological. There is good physiological evidence to back this up. The altered physiology of labour related to the relaxation of the pelvic floor (Sartore *et al.* 2003) results in a longer second stage, a fall in endogenous oxytocin (Rahm *et al.* 2002) and the need for augmentation, a reduction in endogenous beta-endorphins (Jouppila *et al.* 1983) that inhibits movement and a diminution of adrenaline needed in the second stage to maximise expulsive behaviours (Neumark *et al.* 1985).

Simkin's (1989) review of fifteen years ago reminds us of another under-publicised aspect of epidurals: the fact that in a significant minority of women (between 10 and 30 per cent), pain relief will not be achieved in the first instance. This group experiences a persistent, localised area of pain that may take up to an hour to be resolved.

Given the fact that epidural provision is now a nearly universal aspect of maternity hospitals' provision across the Western world, it is surprising to discover that its effect on bonding and adjustment to motherhood has never been studied. There is a possibility of an effect when considering the importance of the hormones oxytocin and beta-endorphin in bonding (Buckley 2010), both of which are reduced by epidurals. Research has shown that putting an epidural in ewes causes them to lose interest in their lambs (Krehbiel *et al.* 1987), but it could be argued that the human brain could counter these effects.

It has been shown that anaesthetists are inconsistent in the information they share with women prior to putting in an epidural. Over 90 per cent spoke of the fall in blood pressure and complication of spinal headache but less than 50 per cent told of the effects on the second stage (Middle and Wee 2009). There is probably, therefore, a knowledge gap for most women about epidurals and during labour is not the best time to be informed. Antenatal education is clearly very important in this area.

The advent of the combined spinal-epidural that mixes a local anaesthetic with fentanyl or a derivative was anticipated as a breakthrough in the effort to reduce the incidence of assisted vaginal birth. Simmons *et al.*'s (2008) systematic review concluded that although pain relief was achieved more quickly and maternal satisfaction was increased, instrumental rates remained the same. Torvaldsen *et al.* (2006) examined whether discontinuing epidural top-ups in late second stage would reduce adverse delivery outcomes, but again it failed to show benefit while it increased pain perception.

Epidural anaesthesia remains one of childbirth's best exemplars of iatrogenesis. It is a wonderful intervention for managing labour complications, especially as an alternative to general anaesthetic for caesarean sections, but has significant side-effects that constantly need weighing alongside benefits.

## Conclusion

Labour pain remains a problem for maternity services and specifically for institutionalised labour care. We need to remind ourselves that research on home birth and birth centre settings on the whole does not express the same anxiety, with neither women nor midwives adopting the pain-relief paradigm. 'Sliding between pain and pleasure' was how Klassen (1998) poetically expressed it in her study of home birth in Scotland. The negative take on pain in institutionalised birth may say more about professional unease. Women's perceptions of pain in these settings are profoundly affected by an environment and ethos of care that critics have described as toxic. Little surprise then that disconnection distinguishes the solutions offered in managed childbirth for dealing with pain. Pharmacological agents strive to mask, subdue, disassociate and anaesthetise by separating pain from experience and reducing it to problem status. I would argue that natural therapies recognise the interconnection of pain with physiology and psychology and strive to work with it. Their health-oriented goals see integration as the path to well-being and, within that, acknowledge the transformative power of childbirth pain.

## Practice recommendations

- Expectations and attitudes to pain and labour need exploring in pregnancy with women and their birth partners.
- A 'working with pain' philosophy should be encouraged and a 'relief from pain' approach challenged.
- Natural approaches need exploring as they have minimal side-effects.
- A variety of complementary therapies should be available as they are unlikely to have serious side-effects.
- Attention to birth environment is critical for reducing the need for pharmacological agents.
- One-to-one care and support from known carers reduces the need for pharmacological agents.
- Mobility and upright postures should be encouraged.
- Opioids and epidural agents are powerful drugs that are incompatible with physiological birth.
- Women need to know the effectiveness, side-effects and increased labour interventions with pharmacological agents, particularly epidurals.

### Questions for reflection

Could you replace a 'pain-relief' approach with a 'working with pain' approach in childbirth education classes and in childbirth professionals' approach to normal birth?

How can you improve local provision of complementary therapies?

What can be done about the rising rate of epidurals in low-risk labours?

# Chapter 8    Rhythms in the second stage of labour

- The medicalisation of the second stage
- Research evidence
- Epidurals and the second stage
- Definition of the second stage
- Time and fetal health
- Early pushing
- Posterior positions in the second stage
- Tips for delay in the second stage
- Attitudes and philosophy
- Practice recommendations
- Questions for reflection

'Push, push, push into your bottom. Come on now Jenny this baby needs to be born asap. That's right … keep it going, keep it going, keep it going. Now big breath in and push again. Come on now, chin on your chest and push down here. Not up here. That's your throat. Push Jenny.' Go! Go! Go! Go!'

Two minutes ago it was just me, Jenny and her partner. Now there's two other midwives, one the soloist leading the chorus and one the echo, two doctors also in the chorus line while setting up for a ventouse, one maternity support worker and me, saying nothing, holding Jenny's hand but feeling I should be assisting with the ventouse. But mostly I'm perplexed as to how it came to this. After all, I had just said there was a bit of delay and the FH was dipping a bit…

I wish this personal anecdote was unique but I know from what midwives have told me from many different maternity units that it is not. Bergstrom *et al.* (2009) published their paper on birth talk taken from their original study (1992) on the second stage and found very similar language in use nearly twenty years ago. I added their description of 'cheerleading' to the first quotation above – Go! Go! Go! Go! One wonders how women delivered babies over millennia without the stern, exhorting voice of the midwife or birth attendants, coaching her every step of the way.

Why does this practice happen? Is it that women no longer have confidence in their own ability to 'do' the second stage without instruction on how to breathe and how to push? Is it that the birth attendants don't trust women to do it themselves? And what are the attendants worried about: is it the length of the second stage per se, or is it possible detrimental effects on the baby or the mother or both? Would the baby eventually be born if the attendant said nothing and left women to their own devices?

Apart from concerns that midwives may have about whether a woman will push effectively, I suspect much of the language around the second stage is a result of a habitual way of relating. How else to explain the rapid assimilation of the mantra by new labour ward staff that seem to know it off pat after a few days? It has colonised maternity units all over the world and has a profound legacy in modern folklore about labour and birth.

## The medicalisation of the second stage

For the origins of the practice, we can return once more to Mauriceau's textbook of 1678 where he gives an insightful description of the second stage of labour. It is worth quoting Dunn's (1991) extract from the old textbook in full:

The bed must be so made that the woman being ready to be delivered should lie on her back upon it, having head and breast a little raised, so that she is neither lying nor sitting for in this manner she breathes best than if she was sunk down in the bed.... Being in this posture she must spread her thighs abroad, folding her legs towards her buttocks ... and have her feet stayed against some firm thing ... that she may better stay herself during her pains ... *bearing them down when they take her, which she may do by holding her breath and forcing herself as much as she can, just as when she goeth to stool...*

(my emphasis)

Is this the definitive origin of the one of the most ubiquitous practices in childbirth of the past 400 years? Probably not, but whatever the origins, Mauriceau certainly contributed to what remains today an aspect of practice incredibly resistant to change even in the face of conventional, high-quality evidence.

In this chapter I will update the evidence in this area and additionally discuss the issue of time and the second stage of labour because the two are strongly linked in the recent evolution of managed, medicalised second-stage practice.

One obvious concern with coached pushing is its tendency to reinforce professional hegemony while simultaneously undermining women's confidence in their own physiology. There is probably no better example of the disempowering impact of the biomedical model on labour and birth than how the second stage is enacted in modern-day birth suites. There seems to have been a widespread collapse in the current generation of women to instinctively 'do' the second stage without professional instruction. When applying Enkin *et al.*'s (2000) two principles to this aspect of care which could be summarised as 'first, do no harm', childbirth professionals need to be able to prove that coached pushing is superior to instinctive, physiological second-stage behaviours.

## Research evidence

Several decades ago, Caldeyro-Barcia's (1979) seminal studies showed that prolonged breath-holding in the second stage of labour decreased placental perfusion resulting in fetal hypoxia, and more recently Aldrich *et al.* (1995) demonstrated that coached pushing involving prolonged breath-holding decreased fetal cerebral oxygenation. These observational studies were added to by two RCTs in the 1990s. Thomson's (1993) midwife-led study showed that if coached pushing in the second stage lasted longer than an hour, then babies had a lower pH at birth. There were no differences between the two groups regarding type of birth and perineal outcome, though the spontaneous pushing group had longer second stages. Parnell and colleagues' RCT

(1993) concluded that coached pushing resulted in a longer second stage than spontaneous pushing with no differences in type of birth, fetal outcome and perineal outcome. On the basis of these two RCTs there is no evidence to support the practice of coached pushing yet it has persisted since. In 1999, an internal audit at a large UK maternity unit of midwives' practice with low-risk women indicated only 8 per cent encouraged spontaneous pushing (Walsh *et al.* 1999). Since that time, I have not seen any published data on this aspect of care.

There have been a number of other concerns voiced about coached pushing from a variety of observational studies over the past twenty years. These include:

- maternal exhaustion (Knauth and Haloburdo 1986, Roberts 2002)
- more assisted vaginal births (Fraser *et al.* 2000, Hansen *et al.* 2002)
- more episiotomies and perineal tears (Sampselle and Hines 1999)
- deleterious impact on the pelvic floor (Schaffer *et al.* 2005), in particular urinary stress incontinence (Handa *et al.* 1996).

In 2006, Bloom published the results of an RCT that was reported around the world, probably because it was published in a prestigious obstetric journal. It concluded that coached pushing had no benefit over spontaneous pushing except in shortening the second stage by fourteen minutes; an interval deemed not clinically important (Bloom *et al.* 2006). Yildirim and Beji's (2008) RCT contradicted this finding of a longer second stage with spontaneous pushing. They studied women who had been educated about spontaneous pushing during the first stage of labour and then affirmed in these behaviours during the second stage. These women had a shorter second stage than those in the comparison group who were coached, as well as better neonatal outcomes and higher levels of satisfaction. Chang *et al.* (2010), using a non-randomised trial method, demonstrated that when spontaneous pushing was combined with upright posture, the second stage was shortened by forty-five minutes compared with coaching and semi-recumbent position in low-risk primiparous women. Women also said they experienced less pain, less fatigue and were more satisfied. The inherent benefits of upright posture have already been addressed in the chapter on mobility and positions (see Chapter 6) so the findings of this study come as no surprise, though the difference in time intervals is startling.

Sampselle and colleagues (2005) in an observational study have classified behaviours that constitute coached or spontaneous and these are helpful in delineating the differences between the two, as there is somewhat of a fine line between instruction and encouragement.

Spontaneous pushing:

- breathing pattern during contraction and pushing is self-directed;
- time of initiating push is irregular (woman initiates push independently, and pushing often begins once contraction is well established);
- pushing may be characterised by grunting with pushing, short and more frequent bearing-down efforts with each contraction, or both;
- open-glottis pushing (i.e. grunting noise while pushing);
- patient follows cues from own body;
- no verbal instruction as to how to push is given;
- no non-verbal instruction is given (e.g. provider does not take a deep breath to provide a cue);
- caregivers offer encouragement and praise only, not instruction.

Directed pushing – following verbal direction, demonstration or instruction from caregivers regarding:

- time of pushing (when to start/stop);
- length of pushing (how long to push);
- position for pushing;
- breathing during pushing;
- strength of push;
- specific direction on how to push;
- instruction to make no noise with pushing efforts;
- actively positioning the woman in a certain way for pushing or verbally directing her to position herself in a certain way;
- vaginal examination with concurrent direction such as 'push my finger out';
- vaginal examination actively stimulating Ferguson's reflex or manipulating or stretching the cervix or perineum;
- following any non-verbal instruction regarding how to push.

Sampselle's study found that spontaneous pushing did not lengthen the second stage.

In a timely systematic review of types of pushing, Bosomworth and Bettany-Saltikov (2006) concluded from the examination of ten studies of Valsalva's manoeuvre (pushing while breath-holding) that the practice should be discontinued because of its negative effects on the fetal heart and on the perineum. In this they are supported by Enkin *et al.*, in the *Guide to Effective Care in Pregnancy and Childbirth* (2000), who state that forms of care unlikely to be beneficial include routine directed pushing, pushing by sustained bearing down and breath-holding.

Apart from the overwhelming evidence over thirty years of the significance of continuous support in labour, I don't think there is one other area of normal birth where the research evidence is so unequivocal. There is no justification for the continued practice of coached pushing and it is probably putting women and babies at unnecessary risk.

## Epidurals and the second stage

The interesting exception to this is women in the second stage with epidurals. A couple of years ago, a group of midwives challenged this exclusion during one of my workshops, stating that if coached pushing was contraindicated in a normal second stage, how could it be acceptable in the context of an epidural when many women's position is compromising descent anyway. The logic of this argument is irrefutable in my view. Actually in 2005, Simpson and James had compared immediate coached pushing with delayed open-glottis pushing in nulliparous women with epidurals, demonstrating that the latter group had better fetal outcomes and less perineal trauma (Simpson and James 2005). There was no difference in the length of the second stage. Open-glottis pushing (pushing without breath-holding) was demonstrated by women audibly grunting, shorter periods of breath-holding (6–8 seconds) and no more than three pushes during a contraction. This is in contrast to coached pushing which involved prolonged breath-holding (>10 seconds), pushing without making a noise and sometimes four pushing efforts during a contraction. In this context, it is good practice to combine open-glottis pushing with upright posture, achievable now with low-dose epidurals.

Midwives may have to adjust their advice to women with epidurals in the light of this information to maximise physiological behaviours, and this probably requires them to demonstrate open-glottis pushing to the women they are caring for. Perhaps at last the ludicrous practice of inhibiting vocalisation during the second stage will then be laid to rest!

## Definition of the second stage

The reductionist nature of the biomedical definition of the second stage of labour has generated more than its fair share of 'doing good by stealth' behaviours by midwives (Kirkham 1999), particularly regarding its length. It is an especially brave midwife who will record the six-hour second stage that included several hours of latency (being fully dilated but without any bearing down sensation). It is far more comfortable to retrospectively assign the start so that the time comes in under whatever the guideline locally requires. Most of us have 'been there' and adopted the visualisation of the presenting part as our reference marker for the start of the second stage.

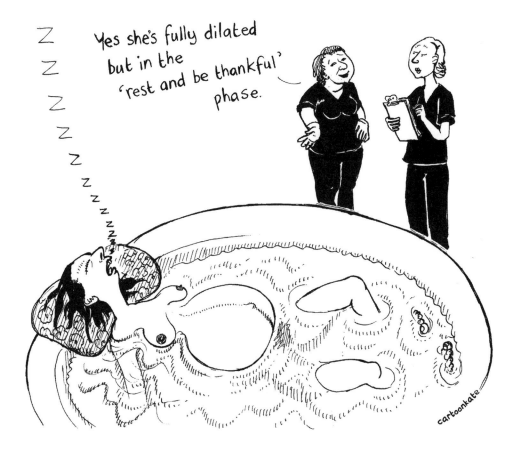

Midwives know that women's bodies simply don't fit the template of the biomedical definition, either because they have a 'rest and be thankful' phase after full dilation or they involuntarily push before. Both of these fall outside the normative physiology. Ascertaining the start of the second stage even with a confirmatory vaginal examination was always problematic anyway. As my midwifery mentor pointed out to me during my training, if there is no cervix palpable on examination, then you are already too late – full dilatation occurred some time before. Occasionally midwives, 'fed up' with the confines of the biomedical model, may deliberately record full dilation at 9 or 11 cm because they argue the improbability that every woman in the world has a cervix that dilates to 10 cm exactly. Of course they are facetiously commenting on the nonsense already spoken about in this book that birth anatomy and physiology is uniform across all women. We noted this rich variety of labour manifestations and timings in earlier chapters.

The artificial imposition of labour stages is classically challenged here because of first to second stage transition: that mysterious phenomenon, virtually ignored by childbirth textbooks (except by the most recent edition of *Myles* [Downe 2003]) and by researchers. Yet transition is one of the earliest observed labour behaviours by students on birth suites and its recognition and care is a key practical skill for the midwife to acquire. Writing about transition more often appears in lay childbirth literature, in books on natural birth and the occasional midwifery journal. This highlights the fact that transition is a 'lived phenomenon', not easily reducible to scientific measurement and not held to be of clinical interest to obstetric researchers. Does this mean that the accumulation of lay literature and a small amount of midwifery writings does not represent a level of evidence, confirming the occurrence of this poorly understood phenomenon? Once again the poverty of a narrow definition of evidence is demonstrated, along with the fact that it is a politically laden concept. The childbirth professionals are the arbiters of clinical significance and they decide what merits researching. For women who experience transition, the notion that it is rather enigmatic and of little relevance would be laughable.

Woods (2006) give an excellent summary of what is known about transition to date and it remains a priority for midwifery research. She describes a spectrum of experiences and emotions (from inner calm to acute distress) that occur in many women in the latter half of labour just prior to the pushing phase. Mander (2002), in an important paper, focuses on labour pain in transition and the challenge this poses for the midwife. It is a stern test of a 'working with pain' approach but wise midwives develop strategies to support women through (Flint 1986), discerning the difference between this and pain indicative of pathology (Leap 2000a).

The biomedical model's delineation of the stages of labour seems to primarily serve the purpose of establishing time frames for each. If time frames take on less significance, then midwives will be freer to work with the lived experience of transition and the second stage and arguably offer better individualised care. The assembly-line imperative is as much in evidence in the second stage as in the first, even more so because labour ward staff seem to believe that they can directly rescue a protracted second stage – hence the cheerleading scenario that this chapter started with. In an overdue contribution on the experiential and psychological aspects of the second stage, Anderson's (2000) interviews with women remain very revealing. Women spoke of:

- the paradox of being in control and 'letting go';
- altered states of consciousness;
- experiencing a sense of timelessness;
- wanting the midwife to be a safe anchor, someone to put trust in, with a calm, quiet, unobtrusive presence;

- unhelpful aspects of care were being treated as a 'naughty schoolgirl', being told off, intrusive interventions, e.g. fetal monitoring, requiring to be on bed, interruptions and being undermined.

Most of their comments relate to aspects of care deleteriously affected by time constraints. One way out of this temporality bind is to adjust the definition of the start of the second stage. Long (2006) makes an important contribution to redefining this by changing the criterion of full dilatation of the cervix to 'when the presenting part has passed through the cervix and is below the ischial spines'. This alteration, she argues, would allow for the physiological variations observed in practice of latent episodes after reaching full dilatation. Once the presenting part has passed through the cervix and has descended beyond the ischial spines, then bearing down will occur as the fetus enters the perineal phase (Roberts 2003) or women experience the 'fetal ejection reflex' (Sutton 2001).

An acknowledgement of a latent element to the second stage of labour and a subsequent lengthening of the time frame has appeared in obstetric journals in recent years (Piquard *et al.* 1989, Fraser *et al.* 2000). Its curious and ironic source is epidural anaesthesia. Anaesthetists and obstetricians became alarmed at the assisted vaginal birth rates with epidurals and at fetal hypoxia associated with prolonged coached pushing. They began researching passive descent, in some studies up to five hours (Hansen *et al.* 2002), before active pushing was commenced. Now it is common practice to wait at least two hours in many consultant units. A blatant double standard exists in these very same units where women without epidurals are only 'allowed' one hour. The perverse thinking here defies any logic. It is safe to permit a woman to languish on a bed, immobile, probably with syntocinon augmenting her expulsive contractions, for several hours if she has an epidural, but not if she is labouring physiologically without drugs, probably upright and free to move at will.

Concerns for the baby when the labour is exposed to oxytocin augmentation during the second stage have been raised by Jonsson *et al.* (2008). They concluded that oxytocin during the second stage is a risk factor for fetal acidaemia after adjustment is made for the influence of uterine contraction frequency.

### Time and fetal health

My own view is that many obstetricians and paediatricians believe there is a direct link between the length of the second stage and fetal health and this primarily drives time restrictions on the second stage. An examination of the evidence, all of it from obstetric journals, in the main does not support this conclusion.

Four large retrospective observational studies have been conducted over the past fifteen years. Saunders *et al.* (1992) examined 25,000 women and found the length of the second stage was not associated with low Apgar scores or neonatal unit admissions. Menticoglou *et al.* (1995) looked at 6000 nulliparous women, some of whom had second stages lasting longer than five hours, and concluded that there was no increase in low five-minute Apgar scores, neonatal seizures or neonatal unit admissions in those women. Janni *et al.*'s (2002) oft-quoted study also concluded that there was no association between the length of the second stage and neonatal morbidity. Finally, Myles and Santolaya (2003) confirmed all previous findings in their study of 4700 women whose second stages lasted up to four hours. Some of these studies found links to maternal morbidity such as infection and bleeding, but these were explained by labour practices or first-stage factors.

Since 2007, there have been two papers that suggest neonates might be at more risk from long second stages. Cheng *et al.* (2007) examined multiparous women and found that in those whose second stages were longer than three hours, their babies were at greater risk. Allen *et al.*'s (2009) larger study over an eighteen-year period concluded that babies exposed to long second stages had lower five-minute Apgars and more admission to neonatal units. Both of these studies were confounded by high rates of epidural in the samples. These studies also showed that maternal outcomes, principally post-partum haemorrhage, assisted vaginal birth, infection and perineal trauma were worse in this group. Some of these maternal outcomes can be explained by compounded effects of more forceps births.

In summary, a long second stage of labour has links with some maternal morbidities but the link with fetal compromise is more speculative. The only qualifying factor in relation to neonatal health is that there is some evidence that when the presenting part is on the pelvic floor, then fetal lactic acid begins to accumulate and this may be reflected in deterioration in fetal heart patterns (Nordstrom *et al.* 2001).

Possibly Rouse *et al.*'s (2009) conclusion is the most helpful in their review of the second-stage duration in nulliparous women. The second stage of labour does not need to be terminated *for duration alone* but on the individual assessment of mother and baby in each case. This recommendation needs to be combined with ensuring best practice in encouraging upright posture and spontaneous pushing, both of which will optimise fetal and maternal health.

## Early pushing

We are indebted to Bergstrom and colleagues (1997) for vividly capturing women's distress with the phenomenon of early bearing down, which was not because of the physiological experience but because of their carers' responses. 'I've gotta push. Please let me push' remains one the most powerful examples of qualitative research in maternity care and a lesson in choosing a paper's title to catch the reader's attention. For a topic where there is such ingrained custom and practice, one would expect there to be a substantial research base. Not only has it not been researched, but, like transition, little has been written about it. This makes it all the more remarkable that even Enkin *et al.* (2000) describe early pushing as a form of care unlikely to be beneficial. In the absence of research, this key evidence source (Cochrane summaries of evidence) felt able to comment on it.

Like spontaneous rupture of membranes at term (vaginal examination is required to exclude cord prolapse), so early bearing down has spawned practices based at best on worst-case-scenario thinking and at worst on myth. Student midwives have been told that it will lead an oedematous lip of cervix which, if left untreated, will slough off leading to haemorrhage. That tends to focus the mind of the midwife: to get the woman lying on her side breathing on entonox or, if that fails, siting an epidural. For midwives committed to physiological birth, the dissonance generated by this is difficult: we are encouraging women to trust their instinctual urges, except in this case.

Downe *et al.* (2008) has scoped this issue comprehensively and surveyed midwives' approaches to it. Using midwives' responses to a variety of vignettes, in 2001 she categorised the midwives' actions under technological, equivocal or physiological. She repeated the survey seven years later (2008) and found a trend towards more physiological actions, reflecting a stronger normal discourse abroad in midwifery culture. Thematic analysis revealed that organisational constraints like time constraints and custom and practice 'rules', place of birth and how midwives integrated their experiences over time regardless of years qualified were all influential in dealing with dissonance. Downe argues for a paradigm of 'unique normality' that incorporates a spread of physiology still within the orbit of normal to address the early pushing phenomenon, as well as calling for more research. In practice, midwives make their own judgements, probably based on parity, concerns about position or strong custom and practice pressures. I have always thought the practice of siting an epidural in the context of early bearing down and/or an oedematous cervix and then infusing oxytocin was anomalous. Surely that just pushes the presenting part harder onto the swollen cervix? Why is that acceptable when a woman's own involuntary bearing down efforts, resulting in the same effect, are not?

## Posterior positions in the second stage

Concern about the clinical outcomes associated with persistent posterior position is borne out by two studies. Ponkey *et al.* (2003) found a link between persistent posterior position and a range of maternal outcomes including prolonged first and second stage of labour, oxytocin augmentation, epidural anaesthesia, assisted vaginal birth, sphincter tears, caesarean section and postpartum haemorrhage. Cheng and colleagues (2006) specifically looked at effects upon the fetus and found poorer blood gases and more meconium, birth trauma and neonatal unit admission.

Simkin (2010), in a very instructive paper, summarised the evidence base of nine prevailing concepts that guide current labour management for posterior position and concluded that only two were proven: ultrasound diagnosis to identify fetal position and digital or manual rotation in the second stage to correct the malposition. The view that the fetus in an occipito-posterior (OP) position will stay in that position is not supported by evidence. Babies rotate all over the place, including from anterior to posterior. In terms of birth outcome, it is the position of the baby at the commencement of the second stage that is the best predictor of outcome (Ridley 2007). Back pain is unreliable marker of an OP position as it can occur in occipito-anterior (OA) labours and not occur in OP ones. A delay in labour without back pain could still be related to an OP position. Vaginal examinations were found to be unreliable in diagnosing and OP position. There is some evidence that changes of position may help OP positions to rotate and certainly many midwives advocate the lunge manoeuvre (creating dis-equilibrium in the hips by stepping up and down, etc.) as well as the pelvic squeeze (pressing inwards on the iliac crests). Stremler *et al.* (2005) showed a trend towards OA rotation in OP labours as well as successful treatment of backache by asking women to adopt the hand/knees position.

I would encourage midwives to read Simkin's paper as well as Frye's (2004) section on OP position in her wonderful book, *Holistic Midwifery Volume II*.

## Tips for delay in the second stage

Midwives have a variety of approaches to deal with delay and achieve a vaginal birth without recourse to forceps and ventouse (suction) procedures. The ones I list here are either experiential, based on general good practice principles, anecdotal or sometimes counter-intuitive, as there has been little research on physiological interventions for this scenario:

- try a variety of upright postures
- consider psychological barriers

- empty bowels/bladder
- offer water immersion
- suggest nipple/clitoral stimulation
- try a change of voice tone or change of carer, if possible
- try recumbent postures, including McRoberts
- try coached pushing but for short time frames
- agree a time frame for these with the woman before initiating an assisted vaginal birth or transfer out of home or birth centres – sometimes mentioning the end point of forceps or transfer to a labour ward seems to bring a reward.

## Attitudes and philosophy

How we integrate experiences that 'catch us out', for example when we encourage instinctive pushing behaviours and later discover a stalled labour at 5 cm, is formational to our practice journey. Over the years authors have stressed the notion of being comfortable with uncertainty in normal childbirth care (Winter and Cameron 2006, Sookhoo and Biott 2002). The ability to not necessarily adjust one's care because of a suboptimal outcome, for example to resist the temptation after the experience above to always do a confirmatory vaginal examination when signs of the second stage appear, takes experience and a supportive environment. You have to be able to say: 'That was the exception and I know the vast majority of the time I can trust the physiology.' It is even harder to hold this position on a labour ward where intervention is common and regular exposure to non-medicated, physiological labours is the exception.

In the second stage of labour, as Anderson (2000) demonstrated, attitudinal change to enhance women's autonomy is imperative because of the history of disempowerment over recent centuries. It could be framed as follows. For women it is a movement from:

- loss of autonomy to being in control
- passive to active
- dependence to independence

And for midwives, a movement from:

- control to facilitation
- dominance to masterly inactivity
- surveillance and monitoring to watchful expectancy
- more to less.

Then the space is made for sensitive, intuitive support that really does make a difference when needed in the second stage as the following poignant story beautifully illustrates from Kennedy et al.'s (2004) interviews of expert midwives. The midwife's account is paraphrased.

> The head was on the pelvic floor and she just said, 'That's it. I am not doing this anymore.' I withdrew and waited and waited. Time passed and nothing happened. Eventually I tentatively said, 'Can you tell me about your mother' to which the woman replied 'Which one. I have two: an adopted mother and my natural mother.' She went on to explain how she sought out her natural mother during the pregnancy and the meeting had not gone well. 'Basically she said to me: you can keep your baby, I never could'. The woman then went on to tell how her relationship with her adopted mother had deteriorated during the pregnancy. When she got to the bottom of that she said: 'My adopted mother told me: you can have a baby, I never could'. After releasing what must have been an unbearable pain, she pushed her baby out.

A facilitatory environment contributes enormously to the ambience required to help rehabilitate the belief that women can 'do' the second stage. Maybe that is why birth centres have such profound legacy in this area. I can think of no better way to conclude this chapter than these words from a woman from society's margins who gave birth in a birth centre in the USA:

> Having my child at the centre means you did it as opposed to a doctor's delivery – if you can give birth you can do anything.... They taught me I could do anything, they gave me control over my body, and that is power: power over my body, power over the government, power over the country. And you take that power and give it to others and so on and so on.
>
> (Spitzer 1995, p. 375)

## Practice recommendations

Care should based on:

- Rehabilitating women's confidence in their own ability to do the second stage.
- Fetal and maternal condition.
- Evidence of descent of presenting part in the presence of expulsive contractions and spontaneous pushing.

- Time restrictions for the duration of a physiological second stage should be as flexible as they are for women with epidurals in the second stage.
- Women should be encouraged to follow their instincts.
- Midwives' role is to affirm physiology, not control it or deny it.
- Routine coached pushing should be abandoned.
- Coaching for women with epidurals should mimic physiological behaviours regarding shorter periods of breath-holding, open-glottis pushing and vocalising.
- Combine deregulated approach with upright postures.
- Transition and early bearing down are part of a spectrum of physiological labour behaviours.
- In the context of delay, counter-intuitive measures may have a place.

---

### Questions for reflection

How could you relax time constraints in the second stage of labour?

How do you approach empowering women to 'do' the second stage themselves?

What is your current practice with women who are involuntarily pushing before full dilatation?

If the second stage could be redefined, what would be its defining characteristics?

# Chapter 9     Care of the perineum

- Episiotomy and its legacy
- Hands on or hands poised
- Other protective factors
- Vaginal birth and the pelvic floor
- To suture or not to suture
- Conclusion
- Practice recommendations
- Questions for reflection

You certainly should not stretch or dilate anything with your fingers. This is a common mistake. This sharp stretching injures the woman's belly (genitals) and causes swelling before the child gets that far and comes forth. Thus the pain of the child passing through is all the greater because of the swelling and the injured belly.

(Siegemund, p. 74, quoted in Dahlen *et al.* 2010)

These are wise words for today's practices around supporting the perineum during birth but were written over 300 years ago. Dahlen and colleagues' paper makes for fascinating reading about the pathologisation of the perineum over the last few hundred years. It also hints at a related issue regarding agency over the body, which is especially relevant for this chapter on the perineum and birth. A hands-off approach to the perineum challenges the notion that a woman's body has become public property for the childbirth professionals. The sense of their body becoming public is reflected in the comments made by some women that labour requires you to put aside inhibitions about exposing your body and retaining 'dignity', often said in a light-hearted way. Yet as Dahlen's paper reminds us, the privacy of the body was fiercely guarded in the past and still is in home birth where no strangers are allowed. Why should it be any different in institutional birth? Does anyone have a right to touch the private places of the body? If there is a need to touch, then who touches and how are important subsidiary questions.

Two papers in the past decade alert us to the assumptions that institutional birth have made about the first two questions (the need to touch and the professionals' prerogative to do so) so that stories of women's pain are about the 'how' of touch. Sanders *et al.*'s (2002) questionnaire on perineal repair found that 16 per cent used terms such as 'distressing', 'horrible' or 'excruciating' to describe the pain of repair and Salmon's (1999) earlier interviews of women found a similar lack of adequate analgesia. In addition, women complained of the insensitivity of male doctors who made little attempt to establish rapport prior to suturing, illustrating the concerns over 'who' touches bodies in birth.

The research that has been carried out around care of the perineum reflects the childbirth professionals' priorities. When the HOOP trial (McCandlish *et al.* 1998) was published, answering the question that had vexed midwives for years (whether hands-on techniques at the time of birth resulted in better perineum outcomes than a hands-off technique), a surprising omission was any attempt to seek maternal experiences of the two techniques. Surely women would have a view of the difference between the passive 'being delivered of a baby' or the more active birthing 'under their own steam'.

The amount of research on the choice of suture material and method of repair represents another professionally led focus that may not have had the same priority for women. When was the last time a woman thanked you for stitching with Vicryl Rapide or for using subcuticular method instead of some other suture or different repair technique? One of childbirth's darkest chapters may well have never happened if women had been involved with its consideration from the beginning: episiotomy.

## Episiotomy and its legacy

Graham (1997) traces the origins of episiotomy from patriarchal notions of the faulty female body through to the surgical mindset of the superiority of controlled incision and on to its close association with the institutionalisation of birth in the West. Along the way, specific rationales appeared from time to time: prevention of cerebral palsy by reducing the time the fetal head spent 'knocking against the perineum', shortening the second stage of labour to preventing anal sphincter tear.

Sadly, the popularity of episiotomy with obstetricians pre-dated both evidence-based medicine and research-based practice so that in the UK in the 1970s, episiotomy became almost mandatory practice in hospital birth, especially for nulliparous women. I suspect that midwives always had some reservations about its use in normal birth but the prevailing culture of the time was to comply with obstetric protocols. An interesting tale was told to me by a midwife who retired in 2002. She was commenting on her episiotomy practice over the course of a forty-year career. In the 1960s, she worked in the community, mainly attending home births, and rarely did episiotomies. In the 1970s she was moved into hospital and was required to do episiotomies on all nulliparous women. She remained in hospital in the 1980s during a time that Sleep's seminal studies revealed that the rate was too high (Sleep et al. 1984). Episiotomy rates for normal birth came down through the 1980s and into the 1990s and so did hers. With a wry smile, she concluded her story by stating that her rate as she retired had returned to what it was in the 1960s, but in between it had swung with the conventions of the time.

What struck me with considerable force was the disempowerment she experienced on entering the hospital domain in the 1970s, such that she felt compelled to comply with a practice she knew intuitively was bad for women. Matthews et al. (2006) addressed the issue of midwifery empowerment in their recent study set in Ireland, concluding with four factors that contributed to it:

1   having control over midwifery practice and access to adequate resources;
2   having support from managers and colleagues;

3  recognition from obstetric colleagues that the midwife's role involved advocacy;
4  having adequate skills to carry out the midwifery role.

From the story above, the first three factors were largely absent from the midwife's tale. Instead, midwives have had to rely on the impact of repeated studies as to the morbidity associated with episiotomy to lead changes in practice. Carroli and Mignini's (2009) Cochrane review concludes that a restricted rate results in less severe perineal trauma, less suturing and fewer healing complications though more anterior trauma, indicating that practitioners are probably simply adding to the degree of perineal trauma by doing episiotomies. The traditional belief that it will protect against anal sphincter tear had been completely inverted with recent studies showing episiotomies predispose to third- and fourth-degree tear (DiPiazza et al. 2006, Gerdin et al. 2007, Altman et al. 2007). In addition, Williams and Chames (2006) showed that the strongest risk factor for perineal breakdown after repair was medio-lateral episiotomy. Finally, there is some evidence that if you have an episiotomy at a first birth, there is an increased likelihood of a tear at the next (Alperin et al. 2008).

This message has been slow to filter through to obstetricians so that the dangerous practice of requesting an elective episiotomy in a woman with a previous sphincter tear is sometimes still observed in practice. A number of papers have condemned this practice (Peleg et al. 1999, Dandolu et al. 2005), including the Royal College of Obstetricians' own 'green top' guidelines (RCOG 2007).

Episiotomy has also been shown to reduce pelvic floor muscle strength (Sartore et al. 2004) and contribute significantly to perineal pain and dyspareunia (Bick et al. 2008), all of which leads Dannecker et al. (2004) to advise that episiotomy indications should be restricted to fetal ones only. I anticipate that maternity care textbooks will begin to reflect this changed thinking in forthcoming editions. In an interesting adjunct to this advice, Raisanen et al. (2010) concluded after their study that episiotomy rates were reduced if induction of labour and vacuum assistance were used sparingly and if spontaneous pushing and alternative birth positions were used more often during labour. Altman and colleagues (2007) also discovered a reduced episiotomy rate in the kneeling position.

## Hands on or hands poised

So many labour interventions have evolved as a consequence of turning birth into a problem to be managed. Inch's (1985) famous 'cascade of intervention'

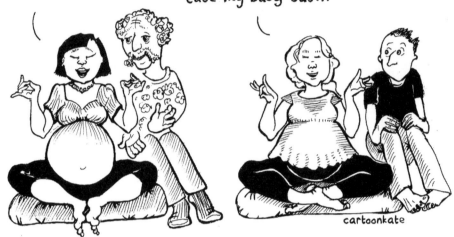

... my perineum is marvellous, miraculous tissue that stretches like a balloon and unfolds like an umbrella. I love and trust my perineum to gently ease my baby out...

cartoonkate

dynamic explains the knock-on effects of taking this approach. Labouring on a bed almost certainly contributed to the epidemic of episiotomy just discussed (ask any midwife how often she has done one with a woman in an upright posture) and the midwifery preoccupation with controlling the delivery of the head by applying hands in various manoeuvres has probably been encouraged by recumbent bed positions.

There is a sense that recent research and physiological investigation has been undoing some of these ingrained practices by showing that non-intervention is as good as or superior to physical manipulation. I constantly return to Myrfield *et al.*'s (1997) paper in my Evidence courses to illustrate this fact. This is not a research paper but is, in my view, an excellent 'evidence' paper. By combining simple mathematical principles with anatomy and physiology, they show that by applying constant flexion pressure to the head as it is born, the underlying birth physiology of extension is compromised. The belief underpinning this practice is that a smaller presenting diameter to the outlet will be achieved, thus potentially reducing perineal trauma. Myrfield and colleagues explain clearly that head extension occurs unimpeded as the curve of Carus changes the direction of force, optimising the presenting diameters as the head extends. No RCT is required to illustrate the common sense of this, though I rarely see the paper mentioned in discussions of hands on or hands off for birth.

The HOOP trial (McCandlish *et al.* 1998), a midwifery-led and multi-centre study, was well conducted by experienced midwifery researchers. One of the less acknowledged aspects of its protocol was the testing of hands on or hands off for the shoulders as well as the head. I mention it because the HOOP trial training video caused quite a commotion when it was shown at a national study day as an audience of midwives waited and waited (2–3 contractions) for the very slow birth of the shoulders in the hands-off technique. It probably reminded them of mild shoulder dystocia, and midwives afterwards expressed the view that this was because the birth occurred on the bed. They went on to say that in their experience, traction was required to help deliver the shoulders when women were in this position, remembering that the diameters of the outlet are not optimal in recumbent birth (coccyx unable to extend backwards).

We return again to the knock-on effects of other interventions like poor birth posture, requiring the additional intervention of physical manipulation to assist what might otherwise be a spontaneous birth. The application of this is regularly seen in standing or kneeling birth where the shoulders usually birth spontaneously without traction and in waterbirth where it is taken a step further by not applying hands to the head either. The question could be asked: is it recumbent bed birth then that led us to believe that the perineum needed to be supported and the birth of the head controlled manually?

Further evidence to support this view comes from the way textbooks have, misleadingly, described the mechanism of labour, stating that the anterior shoulder passes under the pubic arch first before the posterior sweeps the perineum. In upright birth the order is usually reversed because gravity directs the force for the posterior shoulder to be released first which some midwives believe protects the perineum. Many have observed the posterior shoulder catching the perineum in bed birth. Textbooks are reflecting the manipulation required to facilitate birth with women in near supine positions. The classic descriptions of vaginal breech manipulations are the best example, contrasting with the gravity assisted, hands-off of active breech births in upright postures.

The findings of the HOOP trial were equivocal, without strong evidence either way. It was interesting to observe the response of midwives to the results. Some who were convinced that the hands-off technique resulted in better perineal outcomes criticised the trial for not examining the impact of upright posture, though this was unfair as around 15 per cent of the sample gave birth in non-recumbent positions. This subgroup had the same perineal outcomes as the recumbent group. They then argued that the hands-off approach was indicative of a philosophy of birth where women gave birth and were not 'delivered' by midwives. As previously mentioned, qualitative methods could have been used to explore this aspect.

Since the publication of the HOOP trial, three further studies have been completed. Mayerhofer *et al.* (2002) showed fewer episiotomies and third-degree tears with hands off in their German study, but these results may well reflect the fact that episiotomies are far more common there. Albers *et al.* (2005) RCT of low-risk women confirmed the HOOP trial results, though they did show that upright posture and birthing the head between contractions in both hands-on and hands-off groups was protective for the perineum. Finally, de Souza *et al.* (2006) conducted their trial in Brazil and their results were consistent with these earlier studies. From all these studies, the technique for assisting the birth does not significantly impact for perineal outcomes, leaving midwives free to choose either hands on or hands off, but they may want to consider the psychosocial dimensions of their practice and its impact on women's empowerment.

More recently, Laine and collegues (2008) in Norway utilised hands on to slow the birth of the head, combined with asking women not to push as the head was born as a strategy to reduce a high anal sphincter tear rate. They reduced tear rates from 4 per cent to 1 per cent, but results were confounded by a 30 per cent epidural rate and a relatively high episiotomy rate (21 per cent), probably contributing to the high starting rate of 4 per cent. Women were also requested to be in the semi-recumbent position, so it is very surprising that they were able to reduce the rate to 1 per cent. This study appears to support a hands-on approach.

In Lindgren *et al.*'s (2011) exploration of perineal injuries in home birth in Sweden, midwives emphasised communication, environment and reducing fear as strategies that were as important as physical skills at the point of birth. Many midwives would concur with these findings, believing a variety of factors contribute to perineal integrity at birth and that it is reductionist to blame specific practical manoeuvres.

## Other protective factors

Antenatal perineal massage from twenty-eight weeks of pregnancy has been shown to be an effective preventive strategy for reducing perineal trauma in a first birth. Three RCTs from the UK, Canada and the USA have shown this protective effect (Beckmann and Garrett 2006) and women need to be made aware of this evidence during their pregnancy. Stamp *et al.* (2001) showed that perineal massage during the second stage was not effective but Dahlen, Homer *et al.* (2007) have reported on the successful use of a warm pack to the perineum during the second stage which reduced trauma in nulliparous women.

Waterbirth resulted in more intact perineums, fewer tears and episiotomies in Geissbuehler *et al.*'s study (2004) and in Zanetti-Dällenbach *et al.*'s (2006) research. Mention has already been made of the benefits of non-recumbent positions (Gupta *et al.* 2004). Gottvall *et al.* (2007) added to this when they demonstrated a link between lithotomy and squatting and anal sphincter tear in a Swedish study.

Two other interventions that have been researched since the earlier edition of this book are prophylactic perineal injection of hyaluronic acid and the use of the Epi-No. Scarabotto and Riesco (2008) undertook their study of HAase in Brazil and demonstrated a reduction in perineal trauma. Ruckhaberle *et al.* (2009) revealed a protective effect from using the Epi-No pelvic floor trainer antenatally – an inflatable balloon that is expelled from the vagina in late pregnancy. But many women and midwives have reservations about the need to train the vaginal wall muscles in the first place and the subtle message it gives out that the anatomy is not fit for purpose and needs 'training'. Similar misgivings may exist about injecting the perineum prophylactically. An alternative approach is suggested in the natural childbirth literature involving visualisation. With this approach, the perineum and vaginal wall are viewed as being highly specialised elastic tissue, exactly fit for purpose. There is no research on this approach but one can see its benefits in reducing fear and increasing confidence.

There are other factors that contribute to perineal trauma in the literature including nulliparity, large babies (>4 kg), prolonged second stage of labour (Dahlen, Ryam *et al.* 2007), coached pushing (Sampselle and Hines 1999), epidural, induction of labour and persistent OP position (RCOG 2007). Some of these are out of the practitioner's control and some may be ameliorated by the practitioner's advice and skills.

More controversially, there has been the suggestion in the past that anatomy, occupation and even ethnicity may play a part in perineal trauma. There is some evidence for a short perineum (Rizk and Thomas 2000, Deering *et al.* 2004) and for Asian ethnicity (Dahlen, Ryam *et al.* 2007) linking to more trauma but we don't know whether other factors may explain the poorer outcomes. There is no evidence for horse riders, ballerinas, rowers, cyclists, gymnasts, etc. being more at risk, although anecdotally, midwives sometimes make such statements. The problem with prejudging whether perineums will stretch is what individuals do about that judgement. Does it predispose to doing unnecessary episiotomies?

## Vaginal birth and the pelvic floor

I deliberately discuss pelvic floor morbidity here because of information that is in the public arena, vilifying vaginal birth's impact on the pelvic floor.

I also believe that midwives on the whole are not adequately briefed about these morbidities and their relationship to birth practices, so are ill-prepared to answer queries from women.

Technological advances in ultrasound have shown micro-damage to the pelvic floor after vaginal birth (Dietz and Schierlitz 2005). However, it is important to distinguish between mechanical and neural damage in this context and even more important to ascertain their clinical significance. In relation to the anal sphincter, mechanical damage (a tear) is visible and accompanied by symptoms: faecal or flatus incontinence. Neural damage, though demonstrable on ultrasound, will not be visible to the naked eye and, crucially, will not be symptomatic. It is misleading therefore to infer any vaginal birth will damage the pelvic floor. Yet there are anecdotes that this concern is driving some requests for elective caesarean sections.

What is undisputed is that an intact perineum in a first birth is the outcome that both women and practitioners hope for. Rogers *et al.* (2008) tell us that this outcome is associated with the strongest pelvic floor, least pain and the earliest resumption of intercourse. In this section, I will examine urinary stress incontinence, bladder damage, faecal and flatus incontinence, perineal pain and dyspareunia.

Surveys over the past twenty years have revealed to childbirth professionals that postnatal morbidity related to birth is more common than previously thought (Williams *et al.* 2007). Urinary stress incontinence has a prevalence of 20–67 per cent during pregnancy and 6–30 per cent after birth (Mason *et al.* 1999a, 1999b). But before the finger is pointed at vaginal birth, it is important to know that it is also found in women who have emergency caesarean sections where the rates are not that dissimilar to vaginal birth. In fact, women present with this morbidity even if they had an elective caesarean section (Chaliha *et al.* 2002). There is something going on here that is wider than just mode of birth, because Buchsbaum *et al.* (2002) has published a study of the incidence of stress incontinence in what everyone would consider to be a very low-risk group indeed: postmenopausal, nulliparous nuns. Clearly there are gender and/or hormonal/genetic factors that are relevant.

What we do know about the childbirth-related risk factors for urinary stress incontinence are that forceps deliveries (Arya *et al.* 2001), prolonged active pushing (Kirkman 2000), multiparity, babies weighing over 3700 g and age over thirty (Mason *et al.* 1999a) are all associated with it, though not perineal tears. With many of these factors, midwives can have little or no impact but the use of forceps and the practice of instructed pushing are two ways they can. It is also important for women to know that most cases of urinary stress incontinence resolve postnatally.

The prevention of urinary stress incontinence is still best achieved by antenatal pelvic floor exercises (Morkved *et al.* 2003, Sampselle 2000) and by encouraging spontaneous pushing, not instructed pushing in the second stage of labour (Kirkman 2000). Recent systematic reviews are unanimous in agreeing that the first line of conservative treatment antenatally and postnatally should also be pelvic floor exercises (Dumoulin and Hay-Smith 2010, Hay-Smith *et al.* 2008).

Bladder care during normal labour and birth has always been a responsibility of the midwife, particularly if the woman has an epidural. Of course, women self-regulate this aspect in a drug-free labour, so it is a little disturbing to observe what might be described as the medicalisation of bladder care in normal childbirth that is occurring in maternity units. This trend is driven by the occasional poor outcome linked to an over-distended bladder being missed in the immediate postnatal period and by the interests of uro-gynaecologists. In a familiar response to a suboptimal outcome in maternity care, rather draconian preventive measures are being put in place to prevent this relatively rare morbidity. These include routine placement of an indwelling catheter in all women having epidurals, ultrasound scanning of bladders routinely on postnatal wards, the requirement to pass a specified amount of urine within four hours of birth and strict fluid balance charts on all women following a normal birth. This is concerning because yet another facet of normal labour is being 'meddled' with. It may also undermine the midwifery skill of palpating the bladder and finally, catheterisation (yet another orifice to be penetrated) always carries the risk of infection.

Flatus and faecal incontinence, like urinary stress incontinence, is relatively common following childbirth, reported in 13 per cent of primiparous women and 23 per cent of multiparous women at six weeks. Some of the associations are well known: third- or fourth-degree tear, forceps deliveries (Handa *et al.* 2001, MacArthur *et al.* 2005) and sometimes ventouse (Raisanen *et al.* 2009). Others are less well recognised: episiotomy (DiPiazza *et al.* 2006, Gerdin *et al.* 2007) and epidural (Rortveit, Daltveit *et al.* 2003). Epidural is implicated via the cascade of intervention effect because it results in more assisted vaginal birth, more episiotomies and therefore more sphincter tears.

Before a judgement is made regarding this morbidity and vaginal birth, like urinary stress incontinence, faecal and flatus incontinence is found in women who have had elective caesarean sections and in those who had pre-labour emergency caesarean sections (Lal *et al.* 2003).

In recent years, the epidemiology of pelvic floor morbidity has been analysed in some depth (Hannestad *et al.* 2003, Rortveit, Daltveit *et al.* 2003). Rortveit and colleagues summarise the research. The contributing factors for pelvic floor repair in later life, in decreasing order of importance, are:

- heredity
- obesity
- smoking
- HRT
- parity
- mode of birth.

This information exposes the myth that vaginal birth or mode of birth per se is a critical factor in later pelvic floor problems and should help rehabilitate normal vaginal birth as the usual route for childbirth.

The view that vaginal labours and births adversely affect women's sex lives is also common. Research is poor in this area, except on the specific symptom of dyspareunia (Buhling *et al.* 2006) where, together with perineal pain, the aetiology is linked to forceps and ventouse deliveries, episiotomy and anal sphincter tears. This targeting of specific symptomology as a measure of sexual adjustment following birth is reductionist. Many women speak of the personal (do I actually want to have sexual intercourse?) and the interpersonal (do I want to have sexual intercourse with him?) as more relevant factors in assessing post-birth sexual experience. Trutnovsky *et al.*'s (2006) qualitative study indicates that it is the totality of pregnancy, childbirth and becoming a parent that reduces interest in sexual behaviours in many women.

Perineal pain has been under-recognised as a postnatal morbidity with 10 per cent of women reporting it beyond ten days (Bick *et al.* 2008). Protective forms of care include the use of polyglycolic acid sutures, subcuticular method of repair and leaving skin unsutured in cases of second-degree tears. Treatment for perineal pain in the early postnatal period has been well researched. Non-steroidal anti-inflammatory suppositories reduce pain in the first twenty-four hours (Hedayati *et al.* 2009) and the application of a cooling gel pad reduces postnatal oedema and is highly rated by women (Steen *et al.* 2000), though the Cochrane review of cooling agents was equivocal (East *et al.* 2007). The evidence is also uncertain regarding the application of topical anaesthetics (Hedayati *et al.* 2005).

## To suture or not to suture

Salmon (1999) and Sanders *et al.*'s (2002) papers on the negative experience of perineal repair may help explain a growing antipathy among midwives and women towards routine suturing of the perineum following trauma. An internal audit in one maternity unit in the late 1990s revealed that 12 per cent of second-degree tears were left unsutured. At that time, there was no research on non-suturing and it would be an interesting study in itself to explore what was driving the trend. It had always been custom and practice to leave first-degree tears as long as they weren't bleeding and the skin edges lay in apposition.

Earlier, the excellent Ipswich trial (Gordon *et al.* 1998) had compared three-layer repair (vaginal wall, perineal muscle, perineal skin) with two-layer repair (vaginal wall, perineal muscle) and found that two-layer repair resulted in less pain, less dyspareunia and fewer removals of sutures with a similar healing rate compared with three-layer repair. For unknown reasons this quality RCT had little effect on practice until a couple of years ago. Why? It had been supervised by the Oxford National Perinatal Epidemiology Unit and was published in a major obstetric journal. Three years later, the famous term breech trial (Hannah *et al.* 2000) was published with an immediate effect on practice. Consideration of the contrast leads us into the politics of evidence and its implementation. I will cover this topic in detail in the final chapter. Five years later, Oboro and colleagues (2003) repeated the Ipswich study in Nigeria and found exactly the same results.

The debate on not suturing second-degree tears at all was first mooted in the early 1990s when Head (1993) published an article detailing this practice in a midwifery-led unit in the south of England. Independent midwives working in London followed with a retrospective audit of women who had second-degree tears left unsutured (Clement and Reed 1999). This was an interesting paper because it sent questionnaires to women twelve months post-birth. None reported any problems.

There followed stories coming out of some maternity units that occasionally third-degree tears were being missed because of the practice: some midwives were not always checking the integrity of the anal sphincter when leaving second-degree tears. Clearly if tears were being left, then there must be a robust examination so that practitioners know exactly what they are leaving. The conditions for examination include adequate lighting and adequate positioning to visualise trauma, which is achievable in non-institutional settings without recourse to the lithotomy position. There are sensitivities around the routine use of a rectal examination to establish sphincter integrity but this may be required and consent sought.

Lundquist *et al.* (2000), working in Sweden, conducted the first RCT examining leaving second-degree tears. Their results showed that not suturing had positive effects on breastfeeding. There were no deleterious effects compared with suturing and more complaints from sutured women regarding discomfort from sutures. However, the generalisability of this study is limited to small second-degree tears only (2 cm depth × 2 cm length). Then in 2003, Fleming *et al.*'s (2003) UK study was published, which examined not suturing more standard second-degree tears. Their results found that there were no differences in pain between the two groups, but that the non-sutured group had poorer wound approximation and healing at six weeks. Langley *et al.* (2006) undertook another trial in the UK, examining second-degree tears that were not bleeding and where skin edges lay in apposition. Unlike Fleming's study, follow-up was done up to one year. Though healing in the unsutured group was slower initially, at six weeks it was equivalent to the sutured group. Women whose tears were repaired required more analgesia in the initial postnatal period. Significantly, there were no differences between the two groups at one year in relation to urinary stress incontinence and resumption of sexual activity. This study contributes to the evidence supportive of leaving small second-degree tears unsutured.

In the same year, Metcalfe *et al.* (2006) undertook a prospective non-randomised study and found that, though reported pain was no different between the two groups, the unsutured group had more urinary symptoms at ten days and low Edinburgh postnatal depression scores at twelve months. A year later, Leeman *et al.* (2007) reported on an observational study comparing suturing, non-suturing and intact perineum groups in the USA. There were no differences between the unsutured and sutured groups except increased use of analgesics in the sutured group at the time of hospital discharge. In summary, there is some evidence that not suturing second-degree tears is efficacious, but more trials and maternal opinions are needed before definitive recommendations can be made. Cioffi and colleagues (2010) have recently written about how expert midwives make decisions around assessing perineal damage, a paper that is especially helpful for newly qualified midwives.

Kettle, a midwife, is responsible for the two Cochrane reviews on type of suture material (Kettle *et al.* 2010) and method of repair (Kettle *et al.* 2007). Her reviews should guide practice in this area. They recommend the use of rapidly absorbing synthetic sutures because they result in less pain, less resuturing, earlier resumption of intercourse than the catgut group and fewer late removals of sutures compared with standard synthetics. An interesting adjunct to these studies has been other research examining the use of a tissue adhesive for skin closure of the perineum (Bowen and Selinger 2002, Rogerson *et al.* 2000). They showed some advantage over suturing. In 2009, the first RCT of a tissue glue to repair episiotomies was published (Mota *et al.* 2009). It revealed no differences between glue and sutures except that the glue procedure was four minutes shorter on average. Finally, subcuticular method of repair results in less short-term pain and less need for removal of sutures (Kettle *et al.* 2007). For additional information on suturing and perineal trauma generally, I would refer readers to Cronin and Maude's excellent review in *Midirs* (Cronin and Maude 2010).

## Conclusion

Care of the perineum in childbirth has a recent history of unnecessary intervention, and current research displays the same irony seen with other areas of birth physiology: it is busily proving the superiority of nature over intervention when this should have been our starting point all along. In particular, it affirms the wonder childbirth practitioners need to retain about the incredible anatomical and physiological adaptations required during the act of parturition, adaptations that rarely need the intervention of assistants. This orientation also affirms the centrality of the woman in accomplishing her baby's birth. We are just witnesses, not deliverers, of that miracle.

## Practice recommendations

- Episiotomy rates for normal birth should be restricted to fetal indications only.
- Elective episiotomy for a previous third degree is strongly contraindicated and should be discontinued.
- 'Hands on' or 'hands poised' techniques should be a choice for women, and their application should not undermine women's ability to birth their own babies.
- Women should be informed of the benefits of antenatal perineal massage.
- Ventouse should replace forceps as method of choice for assisted vaginal delivery.
- Pelvic floor exercises should be encouraged antenatally and postnatally.
- Leaving skin unsutured following repair of second-degree tear should be an option for women.
- More research is needed on the outcomes associated with non-suturing of second-degree tears of the perineum.
- Continuous subcuticular suturing technique should be adopted by midwives when repairing the perineum.
- Rapidly absorbable synthetic suture materials should replace catgut for use in perineal repair.
- NSAIDs are treatment of choice for perineal trauma and perineal pain.

**Questions for reflection**

Do any of the practices around care of the perineum need reviewing where you work?

How could you counter disinformation about vaginal birth and its effects on the pelvic floor?

Are you promoting antenatal perineal massage?

Is your care for perineal trauma evidence-based regarding leaving skin and small tears unsutured, type of sutures, method and treatment of trauma and pain?

# Chapter 10   **Rhythms in the third stage of labour**

- History of uterotonics
- Components of active and physiological third-stage care
- The RCTs on active or physiological management
- More recent research in midwifery-led environments
- Defining a benchmark for PPH
- Physiological third stage and maternal physiology
- Physiological third stage and neonatal transition
- Language games
- Choice, skills, beliefs and institutional constraints
- Practice recommendations
- Questions for reflection

A midwife, reflecting on current attitudes to the third stage of labour, shared the following story in a seminar. She had begun her career working with home birth in the 1960s. She clearly remembers saying to women after the baby was born: 'I'll just go and make a cup of tea. Call me back when the afterbirth comes out.' Other midwives present expressed surprise that she would leave the woman alone with the placenta undelivered, something many of us were told during our midwifery training never to do. After all, as we were constantly reminded: this was the most dangerous element of childbirth. Many of us remember graphic colour pictures from maternity care textbooks of severe post-partum haemorrhages. The midwife clearly did not have the same suspicion of the third stage. She was operating out of a different paradigm where physiologi-cal third stage was part of normal birth. Was she being irresponsible?

The third stage of labour presents the ultimate challenge to the advocates of birth physiology because this is the area where active management is routinely practised. Farrar *et al.*'s survey (2009) revealed that 73 per cent of midwives in the UK reported 'always or usually' using active management. Winter and col-leagues' (2007) Europe-wide survey found that twelve countries used prophy-lactic oxytocics between 72 and 100 per cent of the time. The evidence base of active management of the third stage has been updated recently by Begley *et al.* (2010) in their systematic review of five RCTs. In a thoroughly considered evaluation of the evidence, they conclude that active management reduces the risk of major haemorrhage (blood loss >1000 ml) in resource-rich countries, but that needs to be weighed against a number of adverse effects. Because of the horrendous mortality in the developing world from postpartum haemor-rhage (blood loss >500 ml), the World Health Organisation recommends active management with prophylactic uterotonics in those settings (WHO 1997).

Since the distillation of synthetic oxytocin in the 1950s, its use in the third stage of labour has become routine in maternity hospitals and we are now into a second generation of maternity care professionals for whom active management was and is the norm. It is against this backdrop that I examine the third stage of labour: the evidence from research to date and the con-textual issues that we must engage with if we are to fully scope this topic. In addition, I will explore more recent physiological insights including Mercer's work on neonatal transition physiology (Mercer and Erikson-Owens 2010) and effects of delayed cord clamping (McDonald and Middleton 2008).

## History of uterotonics

Ergot was first described in 1582 but its use was discontinued in 1828 except for postpartum haemorrhage because of the deaths of mothers and babies, principally due to uterine rupture. The inability to distil the drug from a coarse organic preparation and thus gain more control over its effects was the main reason for this. In the early twentieth century, more accurate distillation was achieved and voices around that time began suggesting that it should be used prophylactically for the third stage (Baskett 2000).

Oxytocin was first synthesised in 1955 and was enthusiastically adopted because it did not have the nasty side-effects of ergot. It became extremely popular to use in combination with ergot as prophylaxis for the third stage of labour in the West (den Hertog *et al.* 2001). Interestingly, RCTs only started appearing in the 1980s so the widespread and routine adoption of uterotonics preceded these.

Ergot preparations are very powerful uterotonics and many childbirth practitioners consider it a nasty drug with significant side-effects to be used with extreme caution. Currently its use is either on its own for the control of postpartum haemorrhage or in combination with syntocinon as a prophylaxis for the third stage. Ergot's unpopularity is reflected in the fact that many European countries no longer use it for third-stage prophylaxis (oxytocin replaces it) (Winter *et al.* 2007), and the UK is unusual in opting for syntometrine (combination of ergometrine and syntocinon) (Farrar *et al.* 2009).

Postpartum haemorrhage (PPH) is a major cause of maternal mortality in the developing world, mainly because poverty and ill-health leave women profoundly anaemic. Millions are unable to withstand small blood losses in labour. The World Health Organisation advocates active management of the third stage of labour in these settings and has a training programme in operation to institute this policy.

Clearly, it is totally inappropriate to argue that physiological third stage should be followed in this context or in any context where women carry significant risks to their health if moderate blood loss is sustained. The key question is: should that apply in every setting?

## Components of active and physiological third-stage care

Achieving consensus on what precisely is active or physiological management of the third stage of labour is problematic to say the least. Widespread variations in practice abound in this area, with a lot of mixing of the components of each (Featherstone 1999). Inch (1988) highlighted this problem over twenty years ago and Gyte's (1994) thoughtful review of research attempted to disentangle some of them. In summary, active management includes the following:

- prophylactic oxytocics
- early cord clamping and cutting
- and/or waiting for signs of separation

- delivery by controlled cord traction
- usually completed within fifteen minutes.

(It should be noted that the timing of the oxytocic, the choice of oxytocic and the timing of cord clamping have been challenged in Begley *et al.*'s (2010) review.)

Physiological care involves the following:

- no oxytocic prophylaxis
- cutting of cord after delivery of placenta or after cord pulsation stops
- delivered by maternal effort and gravity
- usually completed within forty-five minutes
- suckling at the breast if mother breastfeeding.

In active management, the midwife delivers the placenta and must disturb the immediate post-birth period to do this. There is some urgency about getting the placenta delivered and referral to an obstetrician would occur within forty-five minutes if the placenta remains undelivered. By way of contrast, the woman births her placenta literally in physiological care and she can be left undisturbed in the early post-birth period. There is a more relaxed approach to time and, if the placenta does not come, referral to an obstetrician would not be considered until at least an hour has passed.

## The RCTs on active or physiological management

Begley and colleagues' (2010) recent update of Prendeville's systematic review re-analysed the same five studies but used a slightly different methodology for assessing bias and a random effects analysis model for dealing with heterogeneity. They therefore came to slightly different conclusions from the former review. In particular, they emphasise the need to weigh the advantage of reducing major haemorrhage in the active group with:

- significantly increased diastolic blood pressure in mothers
- after pains
- use of analgesia
- more women returning to hospital with bleeding.

In addition, they noted a lower birth weight in their babies, presumably because of early cord clamping.

In separate sub-analysis, though overall numbers were low, there was no statistically significant increase in major haemorrhage in women at low risk of bleeding. This is potentially a very important finding because proponents of physiological third stage have been arguing for years that the trials have not addressed this subgroup which is, of course, of special interest to midwives.

Begley *et al.* (2010) do suggest that if oxytocin only was the uterotonic of choice and the timing of cord clamping and the administration of a uterotonic was delayed, then many of these adverse outcomes might be reduced or eliminated. They call for trials to address these components.

Already we know something about these changes as three further Cochrane reviews address them. McDonald *et al.*'s (2006) systematic review of six trials compared oxytocin (either five units or ten units) with an ergometrine/oxytocin (syntometrine) combination. They found that syntometrine was associated with a significant reduction of PPH compared with oxytocin five units, though less so with oxytocin ten units. Once the threshold of one litre was used, differences disappeared. Syntometrine caused more nausea, vomiting and raised blood pressure. McDonald and Middleton's (2008) review of the timing of umbilical cord clamping found no difference in haemorrhage rates between immediate and delayed clamping (defined as 2–3 minutes after birth), although there was more need for phototherapy in this group. Finally Soltani *et al.* (2010) examined the timing of oxytocin (before or after the expulsion of the placenta) and concluded it has no impact on haemorrhage rates. They speculated that the later timing would reduce the risk of hyper-transfusion to the neonate and potentially reduce the risk of retained placenta, though the trials were too small to show any difference in this latter outcome. Overall, the studies were small with significant heterogeneity and they call for further studies.

In the developing world context, Gulmezoglu and colleagues (2006) examined studies involving misoprostol, a prostaglandin which has the advantage of being stable in warmer temperatures, oral in preparation and inexpensive (and therefore more suitable in the developing world) compared with conventional injectible uterotonic. Misoprostol was less effective for controlling blood loss in excess of one litre and had dose-related side-effects of shivering and raised temperature.

In summary, the trial evidence is pointing us towards being more selective about active management and to revising traditions around the timing of oxytocin administration and cord clamping.

## More recent research in midwifery-led environments

In the last two years, three studies have been published that add weight to the contention that physiological third stage is safe in midwifery-led settings and even desirable in this context.

As has already been noted, active management is so ubiquitous in the developed world that only a few settings where midwifery-led models are mainstream is there a sufficient prevalence of physiological third stage to study its effects. One of these is New Zealand and in 2009, Dixon *et al.* published a retrospective analysis of over 30,000 women in a five-year period. Forty-eight per cent of these women (n = 16,238) experienced a physiological third stage, an extraordinary number. Blood loss amounts were lower in this group at both thresholds of up to 500 ml and up to 1000 ml. In the Netherlands, another setting known for midwifery-led models, no difference in PPH rate was found between low-risk nulliparous women who received active or physiological care in Bais *et al.*'s (2004) study. Fahy and partners (2010) undertook a retrospective cohort study of a small number of women in an Australian birth centre setting, concluding that active management actually predisposed to PPH at all thresholds between 500 and 1500 ml.

These studies are the first that tell us that women who are at low obstetric risk and labour physiologically during the first and second stage appear to complete a physiological third stage safely, and may even be exposed to less risk of PPH.

## Defining a benchmark for PPH

The discussion that follows here therefore is premised on healthy women having babies in the developed world, attended by midwives. In this specific context, there is space to debate what constitutes a meaningful definition of PPH and whether, as Begley and colleagues (2010) speculate, active management should always be recommended for these women.

Critics of maternity care's tradition in fixing haemorrhage at a specific volume that can be universally applied argue that in no other medical speciality does this occur. No operating theatre has set a threshold for what constitutes haemorrhage so that anaesthetists become extra-vigilant once that marker has been crossed. Accident and Emergency departments, where blood loss from trauma is common, have no such threshold. In all these situations, clinicians are trusted to institute appropriate resuscitation based on clinical features, observable blood loss and the specific context of illness or injury. The traditional definition of PPH acknowledges this point by stating that any amount of blood loss with signs of pathology should be treated.

Arguments against setting an arbitrary volume include under-recognition of clinical significance if the threshold has not been reached and over-treatment if it has. There is some anecdote surrounding the latter where if an emergency call is made and a 'skill drill' implemented, a woman is confronted with a team of strangers inserting multiple intravenous lines, a urinary catheter, administering uterotonic drugs and oxygen, even though her vital signs and pallor are normal and, when she gets a chance to speak, says, 'I'm fine actually'. Bose *et al.* (2006) make the point that the altered haemodynamic state of pregnancy makes vital signs measurements less reliable, suggesting that a fall in blood pressure may occur much later than in the non-pregnant state. However, they also acknowledge that the extra circulating blood volume acts as a vascular reserve. Therefore healthy women with normal labours can tolerate a blood loss of around 1000 ml without decompensating.

The threshold of 1000 ml is discussed in the Cochrane reviews as a more robust marker for healthy women and, in the past, authors had suggested changing the figure to this amount (Bloomfield and Gordon 1990). Currently, some maternity care settings have altered their PPH definition to one litre to reflect what they perceive as a more robust marker of pathology.

## Physiological third stage and maternal physiology

Advocates for physiological labour have sought to explore and explain why maternal physiology should apparently expel more blood in the immediate post-birth period. Harris (2001) suggests that the process of returning to the pre-pregnant physiology, which haemodynamically means reducing the circulating blood volume, commences immediately after the birth. Wickham (1999) speculates that active management postpones the passage of blood per vagina to heavier lochia on days two and three and, if total blood loss could be compared between active and physiological methods at three days, the amounts would be very similar. In other words, both authors believe that the extra circulating blood has to be excreted – it is just the timing that differs according to third-stage care. This has not been empirically investigated but there is a certain intuitive appeal to this rationale.

Buckley (2005) writes that the extra bleeding of physiological care cleanses the uterine cavity, flushing out the placenta in the process. This cleansing action of bleeding is a type of ablution that has cultural meaning in some societies. If bleeding assists the birth of the placenta, then it seems probable that active management, where bleeding is reduced, would result in more retained placentas. A possible explanation for this is that early cord clamping results in blood being trapped in the placental body causing baulking. Detachment from the uterine wall is then more difficult. However, only one trial of active management revealed more retained placentas (Begley 1990). It is worth noting, though, that a variation on active management – unclamping the maternal end to allow drainage of blood after severing the cord – may reduce the incidence of retained placenta (Soltani *et al.* 2006).

This practice mimics to some extent physiological care where blood continues to flow, via the cord, out of the placental body after birth.

The benefits of immediate skin-to-skin contact at birth have now been established. Moore *et al.*'s (2007) systematic review of early skin-to-skin contact showed benefits on duration of breastfeeding, mother–infant attachment, less infant crying and cardio-respiratory stability. Emotional connection was fostered by early skin-to-skin contact in Finigan and Davies' (2005) qualitative research on women's experience. Physiological care overtly prioritises skin-to-skin because breastfeeding is integral to the method. The mother–baby connection is not disrupted by any actions of the birth attendant who can simply retire to the background after the birth. Active management does compromise immediate skin-to-skin contact a little. The cord has to be cut and the placenta delivered by controlled cord traction, all within minutes of the birth. This may require the mother to move to a bed and a semi-recumbent position and this further disturbs skin-to-skin time.

## Physiological third stage and neonatal transition

Cord issues dominate recent thinking on neonatal transition physiology. Rabe *et al.* (2006) found that delaying cord clamping up to two minutes in preterm infants was associated with less need for transfusion and less intraventricular haemorrhage. These babies may also be less prone to respiratory distress syndrome. Delaying the clamping of the cord in term infants can provide an additional 30 per cent extra blood and up to 60 per cent more red blood cells (McDonald and Middleton 2008). This enables the baby to start extra-uterine life with peak haematocrit, haemoglobin and ferretin levels (Eichenbaum-Pikser and Zasloff 2009), less anaemia (Hutton and Hassan 2007), better perfusion of vital organs, better cardiopulmonary adaptation and increased duration of breastfeeding (Mercer 2001).

Mercer and Skovgaard (2002) in particular have championed the cause of delayed cord clamping, elaborating on a new paradigm of neonatal transition physiology. Their hypothesis is that a successful neonatal transition is dependent upon a newborn having an adequate blood volume to recruit the lung for respiratory function through capillary erection and an adequate red cell volume to provide enough oxygen delivery to stimulate and maintain respiration. The transition to respiratory independence in this paradigm is more gentle and unhurried, unlike the abrupt eliciting of vigorous respiratory effort within one minute of the birth as is currently practised. This adequate blood volume is transfused from the placenta via the cord and is usually complete within three minutes of birth. The old paradigm held that a robust respiratory response needed to be triggered by powerful external sensory stimuli like temperature, touch, sight and sound coupled with chest wall recoil on delivery. Mercer argues that these immediate crying efforts are not effective at gaseous exchange within the lungs because blood flow has not had time to initiate capillary erection. Not only that but early cord clamping reduces the effectiveness of this stage as blood transfer is abruptly cut off.

Mercer and Skovgaard recall that mammalian birth always includes a rest period after the birth when the cord is left alone. It is only in human birth of recent times that this period has been interfered with. Within this model the one-minute Apgar score is not useful for assessing respirations because this may take up to three minutes to be established. Current practice with water-birth illustrates Mercer and Skovgaard's model as physiological third-stage care, coupled with a no-touch technique and a warm water medium, combine to make babies often peaceful and quiet at birth.

With this new paradigm in mind, there is a sense in which cutting the cord early and effectively starving the baby of oxygen seems an unnecessarily aggressive and harsh method of facilitating neonatal transition and of welcoming a new baby.

What follows from both Mercer and Rabe's papers is that the practice of cutting the cord on a 'flat' baby so that resuscitation can take place on a resuscitaire should be challenged. It makes no sense at all to cut this lifeline when the baby is already compromised. In this situation the placenta is a resuscitative organ and it should be harnessed for this purpose.

Finally, Odent (2002) and Buckley (2005) both stress the importance of not disturbing the immediate post-birth period (more easily achieved with physiological care) when optimum hormonal conditions exist for bonding of mother and child. Endorphins are at high levels in both mother and baby, contributing to the baby's alertness and the mother's attentiveness. In the mother, an oxytocin surge is triggered to contract the uterus and help separate the placenta. This surge is augmented by skin-to-skin contact and breast-suckling. The drop in circulating catecholamines at birth facilitates oxytocin secretion which is more likely to be inhibited if the immediate post-birth period is disturbed and hurried. Aside from active management's imperative to get the placenta delivered, larger maternity units have time pressures on birthing rooms. The post-birth tasks of checking, weighing, administering drugs and dressing the baby all have to be completed, along with readying the mother for transfer out. The 'luxury' of allowing an undisturbed 30–60 minutes' post-birth bonding time would be difficult to achieve. Yet we don't really know the short- and long-term impact of this processing approach for the mother and baby, though we glimpse the 'rightness' of leaving them alone to establish connection at their own pace at home birth.

In the past couple of years, no one has championed the cause of physiological third stage better than Fahy and colleagues in Australia. Commencing with a telling critique of the previous Cochrane review (Fahy 2009), they have mapped out a comprehensive approach to a total package of care in this area that addresses the environment, the midwives' role and the centrality of women's agency (Hastie and Fahy 2009). I would urge all midwives to read this important paper.

### Language games

There is clearly a different meaning attributed to 'haemorrhage' and 'bleeding', and childbirth practitioners use them in shaping women's choices. A colleague was reflecting on this recently and related how the discussion may go during early labour when labour choices are being reviewed. On the one hand: 'There is chance of haemorrhage if we just let the third stage happen naturally. With the injection, it will be quicker and cleaner.' Or: 'If the rest of the labour is normal, it is worth considering a normal third stage. There may be a little more bleeding but you can have uninterrupted time with your baby and no drugs.'

There is no doubt that 'haemorrhage' conjures up risk and fear. The spectre of third-stage haemorrhage is indelibly imprinted into the psyche of midwives

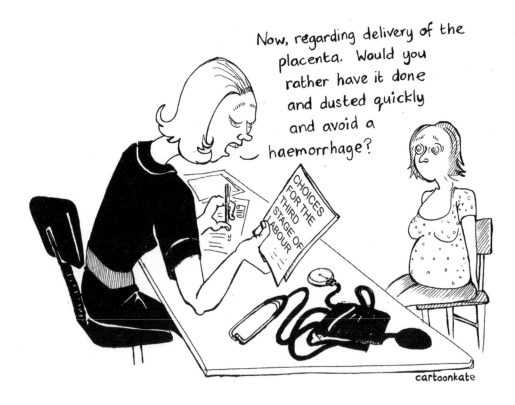

and obstetricians of recent generations. Its alignment with a physiological third stage and the fact that a midwife can practise for years without ever seeing a physiological third stage serves to reinforce the stereotype. Practising in very large maternity units also reinforces it because one inevitably hears of the worst episodes of PPH. This does not cause us to ask the question, 'Why did that occur with an active third stage?' but instead to say, 'how much worse it would have been if no oxytocic had been used'. Many of us have suffered from Wagner's (2001) 'fish can't see water' syndrome in relation to the third stage. It is difficult to imagine that physiological third stage has anything going for it until you see one. As one midwife commented:

> I thought for sure it would take longer and there would be more bleeding but then, after I had attended a few, I found that some were actually shorter and had less bleeding than active management. I felt I'd been conned a little.

## Choice, skills, beliefs and institutional constraints

If physiological third stage remains the pariah of labour care, then the skills to assist women if they choose it will disappear (Fry 2007b), not unlike vaginal breech birth skills. Countries that have enshrined midwifery-led models as the mainstay of their maternity care and home birth and birth centres are the contexts and settings where it is still regularly practised. Here it is undertaken following on from physiological first and second stages of labour in women who are at low obstetric risk. Midwives carry oxytocic drugs for use in these places if required, which is surely the crucial point. Nobody is undertaking this form of care without the backup of oxytocics. If bleeding is unacceptably high, they will be used.

The skills are amenable to workshop-based learning, but there is no substitute for observing physiological third stage which also assists in dealing with the ingrained pessimism and distrust of it as a normal bodily process in childbirth. Childbirth professionals don't own the placenta and its method of birth should not be appropriated by us. Sometimes the institutionalisation of a practice distracts us from these broader considerations. This was demonstrated graphically by a story of a woman requesting a lotus birth, part of which involves leaving the cord intact until it naturally separates and taking the placenta home on discharge (Crowther 2006). When she was admitted in early labour, the midwife, fearing infection and a smelly placenta being trailed around the postnatal ward, tried to talk her out of it, without success. From there a succession of people attempted the same, including senior midwifery, obstetric and neonatal staff. Eventually, the infection control and health and safety departments got involved but the woman refused to change her birth plan. On day two the cord separated without smell, infection or any other nasty sequelae predicted by the hospital professionals.

If a maternity unit has a policy of recommending an active third stage of labour, then it also needs to be able to care for women who don't want this option. This will require it to address the complexities of skill deficits, attitudinal suspicion and institutional constraints surrounding physiological third stage. It opens up the possibility of rehabilitating this form of care as normative for normal birth in women who are healthy and at low obstetric risk. Something of the 'specialness' of an undisturbed immediate post-birth period may then be recaptured from which we may all benefit.

## Practice recommendations

- Women should be encouraged to consider the physiological approach antenatally.
- Research evidence needs contextualising in relation to:
  - the fact that all studies have been carried out in hospitals
  - the historical legacy regarding 'haemorrhage' and time pressure
  - the medicalisation of childbirth.
- Midwives need re-skilling in physiological care, including an awareness of the environment remaining undisturbed and an enabling approach to women birthing their own placenta.
- A physiological approach is the appropriate care when labour is normal.
- If an active approach is chosen, then syntocinon ten units is the uterotonic of choice.
- Cord clamping in active management should be delayed for at least two minutes.
- There may be advantages in delaying the administration of a uterotonic until after the birth of the placenta, but this requires more research.

### Questions for reflection

How could you change the perception of the physiology of the third stage where you work so that it is viewed as normal for normal labour?

How would you ensure midwives are competent in physiological third-stage care?

What should be done about the current definition of PPH?

Is there a need to review early clamping and cutting of the cord where you work?

# Chapter 11 Water immersion and waterbirth

- Environment
- Therapeutic benefits
- Physiological benefits
- Psychosocial benefits
- Professional aspects
- Practical skills for water immersion and waterbirth
- Conclusion
- Questions for reflection

If there is one aspect of midwifery practice that seems to encapsulate and reinforce physiological labour and birth, it is waterbirth. I used this term to include water immersion for labour and/or giving birth in water. It was introduced into UK labour wards in the late 1980s after publicity from the Pithiers unit in France where Michel Odent practised. My memory of it goes back further to a book I read in the late 1970s by Leboyer, *Birth without Violence*. At the same time a Russian boat builder and visionary began promoting waterbirth in the Soviet Union. He became convinced of the benefits of water immersion as a means of maximising physiological potential, and his story is told by Sidenbladh (1983). These books have even greater resonance now as the spectre of obstetric violence gets fresh exposure in journals. In the USA, Goer (2010) has noted how concerns with maternal rights in childbirth that were expressed in the 1950s persist with the current failure to provide one-to-one care in labour, and an undermining of women's choice in labour decisions. Venezuela became the first country to legislate to outlaw obstetric violence, targeting the recourse to medical interventions like caesarean sections without properly informed consent (D'Gregorio 2010). Both of these elements of care should be fundamental human rights because the evidence of their benefits has been comprehensively established (Hodnett *et al.* 2009, Kirkham 2004).

Against this backdrop, waterbirth conjures up the most gentle of entrances for a new life, and in this chapter I want to explore its evidence base to date for a range of labour and birth aspects. These can be divided into environmental, therapeutic, physiological, psychological and professional.

## Environment

There is no doubt that birthing pools contribute to a helpful environmental ambience for birth. You only have to read Maude and Foureur's (2007) stories of women using water to see the effect. These narratives referred to a water immersion facility as a 'sanctuary'. Almost all UK maternity services (95 per cent) have water immersion facilities (Healthcare Commission 2007), with some having this capability in every birth room. Over a decade ago a phenomenological exploration of women's experiences of using water immersion during labour found that women believed water immersion helped them retain control (Hall and Holloway 1998). This could be related to the fact that women usually experience minimal disturbance while there. Anecdotal evidence from busy labour wards suggests that when a woman is in the pool, there is less traffic in and out of the birth room. Is this because she is often naked in the water or is it because the lights may be dimmed?

Either way, other staff seem less inclined to enter the room. It feels like an intrusion into something private.

An aquatic theme is recurrent in newer initiatives around a facilitatory birth space. From Hauck *et al.*'s (2008) Snoezelen rooms to Hodnett *et al.*'s (2009) ambient clinical environment, water, if not for deep immersion, is used either visually or with an auditory component. For the baby, the water medium is natural after gestating within the amniotic sac. The primitive diving reflex protects the uncompromised neonate against inhalation (Johnson 1996). Waterbirth babies tend not to cry immediately they are born and many babies born into water appear more settled in the hours after birth. It is usual not to rush the baby to the water surface but to gently ease her/him up to the open air. Then follows another undisturbed period where the baby is cradled in the mother's arms within the birthing pool.

Thus water immersion and waterbirth creates an ambient environment for all birth room personnel.

## Therapeutic benefits

The water medium facilitates the movement and posture change so necessary for normal labour progression and birth. Stark *et al.*'s (2008) small study demonstrated this with women moving more often and having more contractions than women labouring on beds. Clearly the buoyancy of the water facilitates this as well as upright posture, and demonstrates the importance of deep immersion in a tub as opposed to shallow immersion in a conventional bath. It is now well established that movement during the first stage shortens labour (Lawrence *et al.* 2009), and giving birth in an upright posture has a number of advantages over giving birth semi-recumbent (Gupta *et al.* 2004) – see Chapter 6. Research studies into water immersion reported a shortening of labour (Zanetti-Dällenbach *et al.* 2006, Thöni *et al.* 2007) and a reduction in the need for oxytocin augmentation (Cluett *et al.* 2004). It is probable that the aetiology of this is the synchronicity between water, movement and posture.

The other consistent finding from water immersion research is the reduction in pharmacological analgesia, particularly epidural use (Cluett and Burns 2009, Eberhard *et al.* 2005). Cluett and Burns' (2009) systematic review included eleven trials of over 3000 women. This links with Hall and Holloway's (1998) finding that women felt more in control when labouring in water.

Results from observational studies suggest that women who have waterbirths have fewer episiotomies, second-degree tears and anal sphincter tears (Geissbuehler *et al.* 2004, Zanetti-Dällenbach *et al.* 2006, Thöni *et al.* 2007). Whether these improved perineal outcomes are related to the practice of 'hands off' the perineum (Mayerhofer *et al.* 2002), upright posture (Coppen 2005) or spontaneous pushing (Sampselle and Hines 1999), all of which have been linked to better perineal outcomes, is impossible to determine. It may be a combination of these linked with the water medium itself.

## Physiological benefits

Posture, length of labour and perineal outcomes all tick physiological boxes around normal labour and birth, but the most striking aspect of waterbirth practice to do with birth physiology is the practice of a natural third stage of labour. This practice has evolved as integral to waterbirth and has assisted in acquainting a generation of midwives, brought up with active management as routine for all women, with physiological third-stage care. In the years that I have been running workshops around evidence and skills for normal birth, a natural third stage of labour has remained the last frontier of birth physiology to be rehabilitated as an appropriate choice for low-risk women. Active management has become so mainstream in Western maternity hospitals that there are midwives who have been in full-time practice for ten years and never seen one. Waterbirth, alongside the advent of midwifery-led units (MLUs), has begun to change that.

Though the benefits of an intact cord at birth are now well known (Mercer and Erikson-Owens 2010), it is the alternative respiratory adaption that is striking to the first-time observer of waterbirth. I will elaborate on this later but suffice to say here that breathing is established much more gently and calmly without recourse to vigorous inhalation and crying as the lung fields

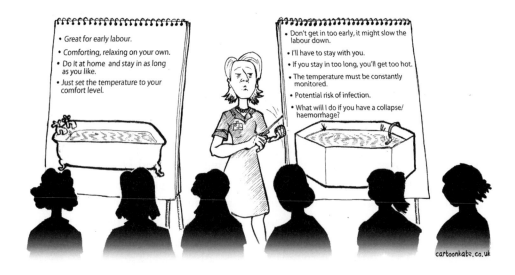

are bathed in oxygenated blood from the intact cord (Long 2003). This can be unnerving for the midwife trained in the imperative of immediate attainment of independent neonatal breathing efforts. It can take one to two minutes for breathing to become established. This factor, plus other problematic aspects of Apgar scoring at one minute (tone and reflexes may be difficult to observe if the mother is the first to touch and cradle the baby, colour muted by dim lighting, etc.), has led to some midwives suggesting alternative markers in waterbirth: eyes closed/staring = 0, one eye open = 1, eyes focused/blinking = 2 has been suggested instead of reflexes (Ening 2010).

## Psychosocial benefits

In the UK, water immersion guidelines commonly require the continuous presence of a midwife, although the rationale for that is unclear. Aside from what is already known about the benefits of continuous support during labour, there are no particular risks with water immersion that indicate the need for continuous, as in uninterrupted, midwifery presence. Some guidelines state that water immersion is not recommended before 5 cm dilated but Cluett *et al.*'s (2004) study challenged the notion that labour might slow if a woman entered the pool before 5 cm. This trial involving nulliparae who had primary dystocia found that water immersion resulted in less use of augmentation and a shorter labour. Access to water should be on the basis of maternal preference and choice at any point in the labour. Arguably, in the latent phase of labour the continuous presence of a childbirth attendant is not always desired or required, and certainly midwives often recommend 'taking a bath' during the latent phase. There is no rationale for differentiating between a bath and a birthing pool for water immersion, though some practitioners seem to make this distinction.

Using a birthing pool for active labour is one way of guaranteeing having one-to-one care in some maternity units but perversely can act as a deterrent, as suggested in a discourse analysis of interviews with obstetric-unit-based midwives (Russell 2011). In Russell's study, midwives viewed water immersion as a luxury that they sometimes could not afford to offer on a busy labour ward. Individual midwives felt guilty about staying with a woman in the pool room when their colleagues were looking after two or three women elsewhere on the labour ward.

However, these concerns aside, water immersion in the active phase of labour usually means that women have access to the continuous support of a midwife if they desire that. It has already been mentioned that waterbirth facilities seem to protect against unnecessary intruders. There is no research on partners' views of water immersion and waterbirth but plenty of anecdotes that they view it positively. Some birth companions will get into the pool with their partner, experiencing an intimacy not as achievable on dry land. I had this experience with the labour and birth of my second daughter and it is a treasured memory.

Birthing in water enables the woman to have ownership of the practicalities of birth because the midwife is largely an observer. Often the mother will be the first to touch her baby as midwives tend to use a 'hands-off' technique in assisting the birth of the baby. Women also 'do' the third stage themselves. There is no research on whether 'doing the birth yourself' is empowering for women but we do know that waterbirth is well evaluated (Alderdice *et al*. 1995).

## Professional aspects

Midwifery attendance at water immersion and waterbirth foregrounds more intuitive care in the sense that 'presence' and 'masterly inactivity' are key dimensions to care in this setting. In Kennedy *et al*.'s (2010) thought-provoking text on midwifery presence, they comment:

> at its pinnacle it is beautiful to behold, but often invisible to the unschooled eye that does not notice or value the quiet midwife in the corner of the room, watching and listening, but letting the woman 'get on with it' in her own way.
>
> (p. 106)

Notions of presence are aligned with paradox. In Kennedy's (2000) own research on expert midwives, she coined the phrase 'doing nothing well', and Leap (2000b) arrived at a similar idea in her study of home birthing women – 'the less we do, the more we give'. The concept of 'not doing' links directly to trust because inaction by the midwife requires her to trust in birthing women to do the work of birth. The Swedish physiologist Uvnas-Moberg (2003) has shown that oxytocin is released within an atmosphere of trust and empathy, demonstrating a physiological rationale for labour progress linked to a trusting presence.

For midwives steeped exclusively in an industrial model of birthing in large maternity hospitals, attendance at waterbirth is about unlearning 'doing' and relearning 'being'. Fundamentally, it requires a reprioritising away from my actions to her actions, from technical to intuitive observations and from time-ordered surveillance to watchful waiting. Observations include the cues indicating endorphin-related changes and subtle alteration in labour rhythms.

## Practical skills for water immersion and waterbirth

Garland's (2010) book is required reading for all waterbirth practitioners. In it, she gives a detailed account of practical aspects of care. Here, I want to mention only a few. A basic rule of thumb is not to disturb the labouring women unless absolutely necessary. For this reason, if vaginal examinations are required, they may be done in the pool. Fetal heart auscultation should be undertaken with a waterproof sonicaid. If the mother for some reason gives birth to the head above the water, then the head should not be submerged for the birth of the shoulders and body, nor the baby submerged if born above the water for whatever reason. This is because of the stimulus that the above-water environment provides that may prompt attempted inhalation. The third stage is best completed in the water as well for the same reason, though some local policies require women to get out of the water for the birth of the placenta.

As with birth on land, emergencies like shoulder dystocia are often resolved by a change of position or simply getting out of the pool. Excessive blood loss (postpartum haemorrhage) is quickly visible in the pool environment. In the extremely rare event that a woman requires assistance to get out of the pool, either a mesh blanket raising the woman from below (cheap option) or a mechanical hoist (expensive option) can be used.

Midwives' reluctance to embrace water immersion and waterbirth range from concerns about rare emergencies (Russell 2011) to limited opportunities to observe them because of a medicalised culture (Stark and Miller 2009) and issues like the ability to maintain water temperature (Meyer *et al.* 2010). As a general rule, this should not exceed body temperature and is best titrated against the mother's comfort level. Having said that, as midwives accrue experience many become strong advocates and, anecdotally, it appears water immersion rates in birth centres and MLUs in the UK hover around 60–70 per cent, with waterbirth rates around 30–40 per cent.

There is no better example of radical increase in waterbirth provision than Durkin's (2009) audit of change in waterbirth practice over two years in a UK maternity hospital. By dedicating one midwife's time (one day/week) to this initiative, rates increased fivefold in a remarkable demonstration of the effectiveness of a practice development project.

## Conclusion

Water immersion and waterbirth maximise birth physiology and the art of midwifery. For student midwives and other childbirth professionals, it is one of the best ways to observe and learn about normal labour and birth. For

birthing women, the benefits are now well established and it is hard to imagine a more gentle transition to extra-uterine life for babies.

On a poignant note to finish, a journal recently published a case study of a
family who chose water immersion and waterbirth in the context of a dev-
astating diagnosis of a term stillbirth (Stocks *et al.* 2010). For them, water
provided the ideal medium to birth their precious baby, despite there being
no precedent for that choice, with local obstetricians and midwives supporting them.

**Questions for reflection**

How could you improve water immersion rates where you work?

How could you improve waterbirth rates where you work?

# Chapter 12  **Changing midwives' practice**

- Relevant generic strategies
- Targeting barriers to change
- Strategies to address barriers
- Diffusion of innovation
- Conclusion
- Practice recommendations
- Questions for reflection

This chapter addresses the crucial but complex question of how to translate evidence into practice. A tale related to me about midwives' attendance at an Active Birth Workshop demonstrates some of the difficulties in this area.

The midwife was responsible for training and development and ran the workshops for three years in a row. The first year she had no trouble filling it, mostly with midwives already signed up to active birth as a philosophy of care. The second year she got all those who were unsure about its merits but were curious after good feedback from the first workshop. The third year she had her own list of midwives she wanted to send but none of them were really interested. Eventually she booked two midwives who she thought would be really challenged by the event and filled the other places from external enquiries. At the end of the two days of intensive discussion and practical skill demonstration, she was interested to find out what impact the workshop would have on the two midwives. One was working on the birth suite the next day and she saw her at the end of the shift and asked whether she was able to apply any of the ideas. Without hesitation, the midwife replied, 'Oh Sue, these women are not interested in active birth, positions and the like … they just want to come in and get their labours over as quickly as possible.'

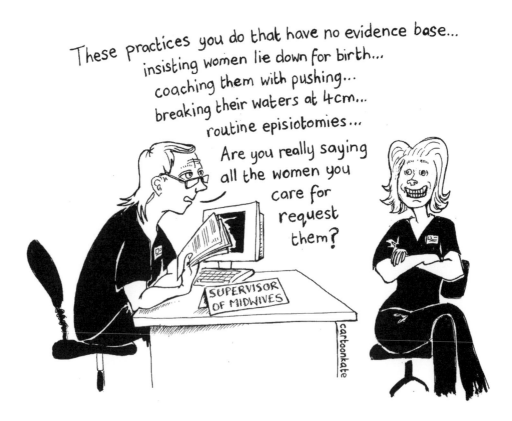

The tale shows how attitudes and beliefs are central to how we practise. If we don't adjust our prior beliefs to incorporate new ideas, then we won't alter our way of doing things.

Because I have taken a broader definition of evidence than just research-informed evidence, I have opened the door to a number of other factors that clinicians may adopt as rationales for not complying with evidence-based guidelines: among them clinical experience, intuition, women's preferences, common sense, physiological and anthropological knowledge, ancient practices and uniqueness of individual women's situations. All of these objections to complying with evidence-based care are valid but there is still a sense that the best research-informed evidence is the most effective and ethical option in a given situation. Even Ann Oakley (1981), an early critic of quantitative research methods, championed the RCT when it showed certain drugs had horrendous side-effects that cancelled out their benefit.

Aside from debates about what constitutes evidence, there are other negative aspects to the new evidence orthodoxy, as illustrated by the midwife who expressed concern after a shift on the birth suite. She was unfamiliar with the new guideline on the post-dates induction of labour. She spent the shift learning how to interpret the guideline, seeking advice throughout the day to this end. On finishing the shift she commented: 'I have not made one independent assessment today but have slavishly followed the guideline. Am I losing my critical appraisal skills and my ability to individualise care?' Or the midwife who departed from the guideline and did not repeat a vaginal examination two hours after an artificial rupture of membranes because the young primigravid woman she was with was doing so well. When the woman had to be transferred later in the labour due to slow progress, another clinician reported her care to the risk manager who contacted her to remind her of the policy. Arguably both these midwives had a point to make about their respective situations.

Much of the evidence around normal labour and birth that we have covered in this book is fairly clear about benefit. But how do you encourage midwives to change practices that are very embedded? The medical profession has been struggling with this question since the advent of the evidence paradigm and, over that time, research has accumulated on the topic. There are six Cochrane systematic reviews and three Cochrane protocols of various strategies to effect professional practice and health care outcomes.

### Relevant generic strategies

Davies (2002) has summarised previous research and developed a taxonomy of least effective, moderately effective and most effective strategies for moving evidence into clinical practice. They are as follows:

Least effective:

- disseminating educational materials like guidelines, practice recommendations and research papers
- attending conferences, lectures (O'Brien *et al.* 2006).

Moderately effective:

- giving audit or verbal feedback on performance (Jamtvedt *et al.* 2006)
- use of local opinion leaders (using peer-nominated colleagues for educational input) (Flodgren *et al.* 2007)
- local consensus process (agreement among professionals on clinical issues)
- patient-led feedback on professionals' performance
- multi-professional collaboration (Zwarenstein *et al.* 2009).

Most effective:

- educational outreach visits (meeting professionals in the practice environment) (O'Brien *et al.* 2007)
- reminders (manual or computerised prompts for each individual patient interaction) (Pantoja *et al.* 2004)
- mass media campaigns
- combined interventions.

(Those interventions currently covered by the Cochrane Library have been referenced.)

When one examines the systematic reviews, the overwhelming impression is that none definitively have the answer to how best to influence practice change and thus the use of a combination of strategies would be recommended.

Other points worth noting are that active participation strategies rather than more passive ones are more effective. The involvement of local clinicians of influence and the mentoring of clinicians as they adjust their practice are also important. Finally, an ongoing audit of process and clinical outcomes that is in the public domain is effective in motivating clinicians to review their practice.

## Targeting barriers to change

Baker *et al.* (2010) take a different tack in addressing practice change by eliciting and then addressing the barriers to change. The appeal of this approach is that it engages with generic change management theory and applies it to health care. The approach appears to be loosely premised on Lewin's (1951) classic force-field analysis model where 'drivers' and 'resistors' are identified. Over the years, a number of 'resistors' or barriers have been identified in research studies and some are common to many practice settings:

- lack of access to information
- not able to appraise research (Veeramah 2004)
- lack of time, poor morale, staff shortage (Hundley 2000)
- clinical uncertainty
- clinical competence
- litigation threat
- patient expectations
- lack of managerial support
- financial disincentives (Baker *et al.* 2010)
- lack of authority/autonomy to change practice (Richens 2002)
- compulsion to act (Grol and Grimshaw 2003)
- institutional constraints (Scott *et al.* 2003).

Grol (1997) classified barriers in another way which is helpful in attuning strategies to address them. Some are related to the individual (knowledge, skills, attitudes, habits), some to the social context of care (patient expectations, professional power, health policies) and some to the organisational context (available resources, organisational climate and structures).

The research has also identified strategies that respond to specific barriers and these will now be discussed.

## Strategies to address barriers

The inability to access evidence and not having the skills to appraise it is amenable to a number of different strategies. Birthing environments should have access to online databases such as the Cochrane Library, CINHAL, Medline and specialised internet search resources like *Midirs* and Google Scholar. Maternity units can have subscriptions to selected obstetric and midwifery journals as, though most are available online, having hard copies makes them more accessible to more staff. Some maternity units hold regular journal clubs and evidence forums for staff. All staff should be entitled to library membership with personal passwords to access relevant electronic journals.

Employment of specialist midwifery roles, for example consultant midwives and practice development midwives, enables them to take the lead in training other midwives in critical appraisal skills, as well as being a valuable resource for evidence information.

Low morale, under-staffing and lack of time sit firmly within Grol's (1997) organisational context and strategies to address these will also be primarily organisational. How care is structured impacts significantly on all three issues. We know from Sandall's (1997) often misquoted research into midwifery burnout that having control over one's working environment, working in small teams and having the opportunity to form meaningful relationships with women all contributed to reduced burnout. Community caseload schemes reflected these factors best, with full-time working in hospital wards the worst. In Ball *et al.*'s (2002) study of why midwives leave the profession, similar factors arose with many hospital midwives feeling disempowered by working within hierarchical structures and obstetric dominance. By way of contrast, I found that a birth centre environment contributed to a sense of belonging and community and an unhurried atmosphere in which to offer care (Walsh 2006b). A survey by Lavender and Chapple (2004) suggested that midwifery-led environments contributed to a sense of autonomy. From these studies a picture emerges of organisational models likely to reduce staff crises, low morale and time pressures: midwifery-led, caseload and birth centre models.

Clinical uncertainty and concerns about clinical competence are focused on the individual practitioner. The development of evidence guidelines for midwives and by midwives encourages ownership and is best a bottom-up endeavour rather than top-down (Spiby and Munro 2010). This means having representation from different grades and experience levels of midwives so there is a sense that the guidelines have emerged from practice. One thing to avoid is having a manager leading or co-ordinating the exercise who is not clinically credible (i.e. she/he needs to be currently practising). There must be autonomy for the group without an obstetric right of veto over completed guidelines.

If new skills are required for the change of practice, then adequate training and support must be provided. Skills around assisting with upright posture, non-directed pushing, physiological third stage or intermittent auscultation are suitable for a workshop format. It is reasonable to expect that those given the opportunity to learn new skills will use them in practice. All practitioners progress at different paces when learning something new, but it is not acceptable to never implement the change when time and money has been invested in training.

The threat of litigation has spawned some defensive practitioners over recent years, with Stafford (2001) lamenting the advent of the 'what if' and 'just in case' midwife. There needs to be a root and branch revision of risk management strategy and operation so that it is premised on likelihood of benefit rather than risk avoidance. As already stated in this book, an explicit acknowledgement of risk acceptance would counterbalance the tendency to worst-case-scenario thinking. A number of small steps could facilitate this, including:

- implementing regular good/best practice case reviews;
- finding ways of rewarding/encouraging innovation and critical thinking;
- a compliments feedback mechanism;
- user involvement in assessing risk;
- contextual risk assessment so that generic hospital-wide applications are not transposed into maternity care;
- avoiding blindness to normative institutional practices that constitute risks to normal labour and birth;
- streamlining record-keeping so that midwives have more time to be with labouring women (Walsh 2006b).

In the maternity care context, patient expectations can be translated as information, choice and control regarding labour and birth options. What is seldom examined here is not what women articulate about these but how midwives integrate and evolve their own values and practices around birth care. We know that institutional pressures generate survival mechanisms in midwives which cause them to stereotype women (Hunt and Symonds 1995), disengage from relationships (Stapleton *et al.* 2002) and practise furtively to protect women from intervention (Kirkham 1999). We get insights into how midwives integrate their experiences with their approach to care in Kirkham's important book, *The Midwife–Mother Relationship*, now in its second edition (Kirkham 2010) and in Hunter and Deery's (2009) edited book, which is a welcome exploration of the affective domain of midwifery work.

Though many midwives are reflective by nature, we seldom get time to examine our values around our practice in any sort of structured way. Kirkham's (1995) personal construct laddering exercise is a useful way into this and can be done alone or as a group activity. Part of it involves brainstorming on one's own ideas and thoughts under headings such as 'childbirth', 'the midwife's role', 'the obstetrician's role' and doing a SWOT (strengths, weaknesses, opportunities, threats) analysis based on your identified aspirations. The self-awareness and self-knowledge generated through these activities or the use of reflective diaries can assist us in caring for women with contrasting expectations and in trying to bring congruence to dissonant clinical experiences. Throughout this book I have explored philosophies of care and how they interface with evidence, aligning the orientation of this book to a social model. In fleshing out how this may impact on the midwife–woman relationship, the following ideas may clarify nuances of this, in particular the movement from a more traditional hierarchical model to an egalitarian one:

- from director to facilitator
- from leader to follower
- from surveillance to 'skilled companionship'
- from neutral observer to advocate/partnership
- from paternalism to mutuality/reciprocity
- from formal and professional to informal and personal.

The barriers of lack of autonomy and authority are often linked with lack of managerial support. This is a vexed question for midwives who work closely with obstetricians who have a legacy of dominating them (Donnison 1988), with links to nursing which has also suffered under medical hegemony (Coombs and Ersser 2004). One approach is to strive to establish midwifery as a primary-care-based occupation. This would require the movement of birth out of acute settings into birth centres, midwifery-led units and home. Though this trend is occurring, it is happening slowly and is unlikely to usurp hospitals as the principal place of birth. There are models across the world that have a hybrid system of community-based group practices of midwives carrying caseloads with another grouping of midwives working alongside obstetricians in hospitals (for example, in New Zealand). Even here, though, the interface between both groups can either be facilitatory or dysfunctional (Dawson 2006). There is reasonable evidence that poor communication and team dynamics adversely affects care in maternity care (Downe and Finlayson 2011) and in wider health environs (Zwarenstein *et al.* 2006).

Strategies that create dialogue between professional groups in a nonthreatening environment are to be encouraged. The ALSO course is a good example of inter-professional learning that has achieved this end. Undertaken away from an individual's clinical setting with a level playing field for all participants and tutors drawn equally from midwives and obstetricians, it sets up an egalitarian context for engagement.

Reverse debates are another strategy for encouraging understanding, as a midwife argues for something she is diametrically opposed to, as does an obstetrician. Learning from exemplars of positive interpersonal dynamics that do exist in some maternity care settings is another way of addressing this difficult and under-researched area (Cheung and Fleming 2011). Finally, midwifery needs to nurture transformational leaders who can run with this agenda and lead by example (Byrom *et al.* 2011).

Grol and Grimshaw (2003) write of a medical imperative that compels doctors to act, to be seen to be doing something when doing nothing might be the most appropriate 'intervention'. This has particular relevance to midwifery where, in relation to labour, watchful waiting may be more important than a constant 'doing' of tasks. As discussed in Chapter 4, 'being with' women rather than 'doing to' women requires some unlearning of an institutional mindset. There is an accumulating body of papers now on midwifery 'presence' and its power (Kennedy *et al.* 2010, Pembroke and Pembroke 2008), with a clear link to having time with women. Temporality and the need to move away from clock time to biological time is another theme in recent books (McCourt 2010) and journal articles (Brown and Chandra 2009). The industrial model of processing women (a 'doing' and 'time' regulated activity) as if on an assembly-line has dominated large maternity unit practice for decades now and needs challenging (Walsh 2006b).

Applications for the maternity service include down-sizing to smaller organisational units like birth centres and caseload-holding, self-managing teams. Valuing qualitative markers like women's experience of care, carers' job satisfaction and the sense of nurture, compassion and community within the practice setting are needed alongside the traditional quantitative markers of process and clinical outcomes and activity levels. As an antidote to the clock-time-driven dynamic of labour care, Winter and Cameron (2006) counsel us to be comfortable with uncertainty and mystery so that our interventions in labour respect its rhythms.

Institutional constraints on evidence-based care arise because a powerful underlying driver to activity is the institution's interests, not those of the patients. These may be the interests of the professionals who staff it or the managers who run it or accountants who finance it. In maternity units there are numerous professional-centred activities and arrangements like ward rounds and hierarchies that have nothing to do with serving the interests of women. Very recently a friend accompanied her daughter for her first birth into a large UK maternity hospital and left with the overwhelming impression that care was set up to serve the institution, not the individual woman. Management interests are served by constant reorganisations and reconfigurations that don't appear to improve women's care and cause long-term staff to say, 'I've seen it all before. They have just given it another name.' The key question is always: how will this serve the interests of women better than the previous arrangement? Scale effects are seminal here as the bigger an organisation becomes, the more the scope of management expands. It is worth restating the differences between large and small scale, listed in the first chapter.

TABLE 12.1

| Large scale | Small scale |
| --- | --- |
| Bureaucratic | Pragmatic |
| Institutional | Homely |
| Hierarchical | Non-hierarchical |
| Impersonal | Personal |
| Formal | Informal |
| Rigidity | Flexibility |
| Standardised | Individualised |
| Control | Autonomy |
| Throughput | Input |
| Risk | Efficacy |
| Organisation | Community |
| Time-bound | 'Go with the flow' |
| 'Doing' | 'Being' |

## Diffusion of innovation

Prior to concluding this chapter, I will summarise one other model of change management that is gaining credence in health care circles for addressing practice change – Rogers' (1995) diffusion of innovation. The theory states that there are five elements that determine whether, in the case of health care, a new clinical behaviour will be adopted:

1 relative advantage (degree to which clinicians view the new behaviour/practice as better than the one it supersedes);
2 compatibility (degree to which innovation is perceived to be congruent with values, past experience and needs of adopters);
3 complexity (degree of difficulty in understanding and using new practice);
4 trialability (the ease with which the new practice can be experimented with and modified);
5 observability (degree to which the results of the innovation are visible to others).

Sanson-Fisher (2004) promotes this approach but then warns of the characteristics of the social context that will be most likely to be successful with it. They are settings with 'a culture of creativity and innovation, a relatively flat hierarchical system and where there is strong leadership that is committed to effecting change' (p. S56). This chimes with earlier discussions here about optimising the social and organisational context.

## Conclusion

There is a natural tendency to be pessimistic about practice change when so much of its success is tied up with issues beyond the scope of the individual. However, we can take encouragement from the fact that over the course of our professional lives we all make adjustments to our practice on the basis of experience and new learning. For some, these may be quantum changes, for others minor adjustments. It is rare for practices to become entirely fossilised and remain unchallenged over decades. One of the most encouraging examples of substantive practice change is the ever-burgeoning provision of waterbirth. Clearly there are many midwives who have internalised this skill over the last fifteen years and that adjustment is considerable, incorporating several changes that form the total package of assisting with a waterbirth. A hands-off technique, physiological third stage and birth in non-recumbent posture are among these.

Bringing about change in practice at a unit-wide level is, of course, more challenging. The best starting point is doing some analysis of the likely local barriers to change where you work and then targeting strategies to addressing these. We can draw on the research findings addressed in this chapter in selecting appropriate strategies.

Evidence-based care is here to stay because it emphasises the best and most effective care in any given situation, given all the vagaries that may be present. As a concept it is already morphing into something much more than just research-informed evidence, and I have discussed in this book a number of additional sources of evidence that are beginning to gain credibility. This is exciting for midwives involved in intrapartum care because of the variability in labour behaviours and Downe and McCourt's (2008) idea of 'unique normality'. The privilege of journeying with a woman through one of the great 'rite-of-passage' transitions of life requires us to draw widely and deeply from the pool of wisdom that informs this area. In that quest we will contribute to the rolling back of centuries of medicalisation that has undermined and discredited labour physiology. We will also assist in rehabilitating women's agency which has been eroded by professional hegemony over the same period. If evidence-based care facilitates the realisation of those twin purposes, then its legacy will be profound indeed.

### Practice recommendations

- When undertaking a practice change initiative, do some analysis of likely local barriers to change.
- Adopt a range of strategies when planning practice change.

- Use bottom-up approaches so that midwife ownership is maximised.
- Get sign-up from known opinion-leader/influential midwives within the practice setting.
- Remember to include an examination of organisational factors inhibiting practice development like reactive risk management, hierarchical structures and institutional 'rules'.
- Use audit mechanisms to emphasise best practice outcomes.

---

**Questions for reflection**

How can midwifery autonomy in practices around normal birth be supported?

How can you cultivate a reflective, learning environment where you work?

How can user involvement in practice change be encouraged?

Could you set up regular peer-review meetings that examine evidence for practice?

---

# Appendix

## Relevant journals for childbirth

APPENDIX TABLE

| Title | Where available |
|-------|-----------------|
| *Acta Obstetrica et Gynaecologica* | Wiley: http://onlinelibrary.wiley.com/journal/10.1111/(ISSN)1600-0412<br>Comment: Scandinavian journal of college of obs and gynae. Obstetric rather than midwifery focus but publishes some qualitative papers and papers by midwives. Research-oriented. |
| *American Journal of Obstetrics & Gynecology* | Elsevier: www.elsevier.com/wps/find/journaldescription.cws_home/623277/description#description<br>Comment: Obstetric and quantitative research focus. Occasional normal birth paper. |
| *Australian and New Zealand Journal of Obstetrics and Gynaecology* | Wiley: http://onlinelibrary.wiley.com/journal/10.1111/(ISSN)1479-828X<br>Comment: Obstetric and quantitative research focus. Occasional normal birth paper. |
| *Birth* | Wiley: http://onlinelibrary.wiley.com/journal/10.1111/(ISSN)1523–536X<br>Comment: Best multi-disciplinary childbirth journal out there. Recommended. Research-oriented. |
| *BMC Pregnancy and Childbirth* | Free BioMed Central; www.biomedcentral.com/bmcpregnancychildbirth<br>Comment: Biomedical focus but increasingly a source of international research papers on childbirth |
| *BJM* | Internurse: www.internurse.com/internurse/Journals/28<br>Comment: Important for UK midwives but carries international papers. Becoming more research-oriented |
| *British Medical Journal* | Free: http://bmj.bmjjournals.com<br>Comment: Carries occasional childbirth research paper, usually of international importance. |

*continued*

APPENDIX TABLE *cont.*

| Title | Where available |
|---|---|
| BJOG: An International Journal of Obstetrics and Gynaecology | Wiley: www.bjog.org/view/0/index.html<br>Comment: Often carries a paper relevant to normal birth and occasional midwifery authors. |
| Complementary Therapies in Clinical Practice (formerly Complementary Therapies in Nursing & Midwifery) | Elsevier: www.elsevier.com/wps/find/journaldescription.cws_home/704176/description#description<br>Comment: a must if interested in the research base of complementary therapies. Regularly carries childbirth-related papers. |
| European Journal of Obstetrics & Gynecology and Reproductive Biology | Elsevier: www.elsevier.com/wps/find/journaldescription.cws_home/505961/description#description<br>Comment: Obstetric and quantitative research focus. Occasional normal birth paper. |
| Evidence Based Midwifery | Royal College of Midwives: www.rcm.org.uk/ebm<br>Comment: accompanies RCM's journal *Midwives*. Research-based papers only, with UK focus. Has increasing credibility. |
| Health Care of Women International | Ingenta: www.ingentaconnect.com/content/routledg/uhcw<br>Comment: Occasional childbirth-related paper. Research papers more likely to be qualitative. |
| International Journal of Childbirth | Springer Publishing: www.springerpub.com/product/21565287<br>Comment: New journal on all aspects of maternity care launched in 2011. Broad-based, multi-disciplinary, supported by the ICM. |

|  |  |
| --- | --- |
| International Journal of Obstetrics & Gynecology | Elsevier: www.elsevier.com/wps/find/journaldescription.cws_home/506037/description#description Comment: Obstetric and quantitative research focus. Occasional normal birth paper. |
| Journal of Advanced Nursing | Wiley: www.journalofadvancednursing.com Comment: High-quality occasional midwifery-related papers, usually research. |
| Journal of Human Lactation | Sage Publications: http://online.sagepub.com Comment: a must for infant feeding interest. |
| Journal of Midwifery & Women's Health | Wiley http://onlinelibrary.wiley.com/journal/10.1111/(ISSN)1542-2011. Comment: American College of Nurse/Midwives. Very relevant internationally with regular and significant research papers. |
| Journal of Obstetric, Gynecology & Neonatal Nursing (JOGNN) | Wiley www.wiley.com/bw/journal.asp?ref=0884-2175 Comment: Relevant and intermittently publishes important midwifery research papers. |
| Journal of Obstetrics and Gynaecology | Taylor & Francis: www.informaworld.com/smpp/home~db=all Comment: Inferior cousin to BJOG. Obstetric and quantitative research focus. Occasional normal birth paper. |
| Journal of Psychosomatic Obstetrics and Gynaecology | Informa: http://informahealthcare.com/pob Comment: Quirky, fascinating journal. Often relevant papers, some by midwives. |
| Journal of Reproductive & Infant Psychology | Taylor & Francis: www.tandf.co.uk/journals/titles/02646838.html Comment: A lesser-known gem that has many research papers relevant to psychological aspects of childbirth. |

continued

APPENDIX TABLE *cont.*

| Title | Where available |
|---|---|
| Lancet | Lancet: www.thelancet.com<br>Comment: Carries occasional childbirth research paper, usually of international importance. |
| Maternal and Child Nutrition | Wiley: www.wiley.com/bw/journal.asp?ref=1740-8695<br>Comment: Newish journal with international scope and research focus. Obvious relevance to midwives. |
| Midirs | www.midirs.org.uk<br>Comment: Indispensable for midwives. A must. |
| Midwifery | Science Direct: www.sciencedirect.com/science/journal/02666138<br>Comment: Top of the league for midwifery research internationally. Lots of fascinating qualitative papers. |
| Midwifery Today | www.midwiferytoday.com/magazine<br>Comment: Small on research but huge on experience and rich anecdote. Unashamedly pro normality. Always something rewarding for midwives to read. |
| Obstetrics & Gynecology | Wolters Klewer: http://journals.lww.com/greenjournal/pages/default.aspx<br>Comment: High-impact factor for academics. Obstetric and quantitative research focus. Occasional normal birth paper. |
| New England Journal of Medicine | Free; http://content.nejm.org<br>Comment: US equivalent of *BMJ* and *Lancet*. Comment: Carries occasional childbirth research paper, usually of international importance. |

| New Zealand Journal of Midwifery | Free: www.midwife.org.nz/index.cfm/1,114,0,0,html/NZCOM-Journal<br>Comment: Latest papers from this haven of midwifery-led care and autonomy. |
| --- | --- |
| Qualitative Health Research | Sage Publications: http://qhr.sagepub.com<br>Comment: All you want to know about qualitative research method. Very occasional childbirth-related paper. |
| Sociology of Health & Illness | Blackwell Publishing: www.blackwellpublishing.com/shil_enhanced<br>Comment: Occasional insightful and important papers on midwifery and childbirth with sociological bent and important critical focus. |
| Social Science & Medicine | Elsevier: http://journals.elsevier.com/02779536/social-science-and-medicine<br>Comment: Occasional insightful and important papers on midwifery and childbirth with sociological bent and important critical focus. |
| The Practising Midwife | Elsevier: www.elsevier.com/wps/find/journaldescription.cws_home/703955/description#description<br>Comment: Very readable and informative UK journal. Light on research but great for practice relevance. |
| Women & Birth | Elsevier: www.elsevier.com/wps/find/journaldescription.cws_home/707424/description#description<br>Comment: Australian College of Midwives. New journal with emphasis on research |

Note
Zetoc Alert: http://zetoc.mimas.ac.uk/alertguide.html (service enabling subscriber to receive contents pages of any journal nominated to be emailed to you).

# Bibliography

Albers, L. (1999) The duration of labour in healthy women. *Journal of Perinatology*, 19(2): 114–19.

Albers, L., Anderson, D. and Cragin, L. (1997) The relationship of ambulation in labour to operative delivery. *Journal of Nurse Midwifery*, 42(1): 4–8.

Albers, L., Sedler, K., Bedrick, E., Teaf, D. and Peralta, P. (2005) Midwifery care measures in the second stage of labour and reduction of genital tract trauma at birth: a randomised controlled trial. *Journal of Midwifery & Women's Health*, 50: 365–72.

Alderdice, F., Renfrew, M. and Marchant, S. (1995) Labour and birth in water in England and Wales: survey report. *British Journal of Midwifery*, 3(7): 375–82.

Aldrich, C., D'Antona, D., Spencer, J., Wyatt, J.S., Peebles, D.M., Delpy, D.T. and Reynolds, E.O. (1995) The effects of maternal pushing on fetal cerebral oxygenation and blood volume during the second stage of labour. *BJOG*, 102(6): 448–53.

Aldrich, S. and Eccleston, C. (2000) Making sense of everyday pain. *Social Science & Medicine*, 50: 1631–41.

Alfirevic, Z., Devane, D. and Gyte, G. (2006) Continuous cardiotocography (CTG) as a form of electronic fetal monitoring (EFM) for fetal assessment during labour. *Cochrane Database of Systematic Reviews*, Issue 3.

Allen, R., Bowling, F. and Oats, J. (2004) Determining the fetal scalp level that indicates the need for intervention in labour. *Australian and New Zealand Journal of Obstetrics and Gynaecology*, 44: 549–52.

Allen, V., Baskett, T., O'Connell, C., McKeen, D. and Allen, A. (2009) Maternal and perinatal outcomes with increasing duration of the second stage of labour. *Obstetrics & Gynecology*, 113(6): 1248–58.

Alperin, M., Krohn, M. and Parviainen, K. (2008) Episiotomy and increase in the risk of obstetric laceration in a subsequent vaginal delivery. *Obstetrics & Gynecology*, 111: 1274–8.

Altman, D., Ragnar, I. and Ekstrom, A. (2007) Anal sphincter lacerations and upright delivery postures: a risk analysis from a randomised controlled trial. *International Urogynecology Journal*, 18: 141–6.

Alzugaray, M. (2001) A midwifery-based holistic prenatal water exercise and educational program. *Midwifery Today International Midwife*, 59: 25–6.

Amelink-Verburg, M. and Buitendijk, S. (2010) Pregnancy and labour in the Dutch maternity care system: what is normal? The role division between midwives and obstetricians. *Journal of Midwifery & Women's Health*, 55: 216–25.

Ananth, C., Smulian, J. and Vintzeleos, A. (1997) The association of placenta praevia with history of caesarean delivery and abortion: a meta-analysis. *American Journal of Obstetrics & Gynecology*, 177(5): 1071–8.

Anderson, T. (2000) Feeling safe enough to let go: the relationship between the woman and her midwife in the second stage of labour. In M. Kirkham (ed.) *The Midwife–Woman Relationship*. London: Routledge.

Anderson, T. (2004) *The Impact of the Age of Risk for Antenatal Education*. Paper presented at NCT conference, Coventry, 13 March.

Andrews, C. and Chrzanowski, M. (1990) Maternal position, labour and comfort. *Applied Nursing Research*, 3: 7.

Anim-Somuah, M., Smyth, R. and Howell, C. (2006) Epidural versus non-epidural or no analgesia in labour. *Cochrane Database of Systematic Reviews*, Issue 2.

Annandale, E. (1987) Dimensions of patient control in a free-standing birth centre. *Social Science & Medicine*, 25(11): 1235–48.

Annandale, E. (1988) How midwives accomplish natural birth: managing risk and balancing expectation. *Social Problems*, 35(2): 95–110.

Arya, L., Jackson, N., Myers, D. and Verma, A. (2001) Risk of new onset urinary inconsistence after forceps and vacuum delivery in primiparous women. *American Journal of Obstetrics & Gynecology*, 185: 1318–24.

Aschkenasy, J. (2003) Sound healing. *Spirituality and Health*, July/August. Online: www.spiritualityhealth.com/NMagazine/articles.php?id=380.

Bailit, J., Dierker, L., Blanchard, M. and Mercer, B. (2005) Outcomes of women presenting in active versus latent phase of spontaneous labour. *Obstetrics & Gynecology*, 105: 77–9.

Baines, S. and Murphy, S. (2010) *Aquatic Exercise for Pregnancy: A Resource Book for Midwives and Health and Fitness Professionals*. London: M & K Update, Ltd.

Bais, J., Eskes, M., Pel M., Bonsel, G. and Bleker, O. (2004) Postpartum haemorrhage in nulliparous women: incidence and risk factors in low and high risk women. *European Journal of Obstetrics & Gynecology and Reproductive Biology*, 115(2): 166–72.

Baker, A. and Kenner, A. (1993) Communication of pain: vocalisation as an indicator of the stage of labour. *Australian and New Zealand Journal of Obstetrics and Gynaecology*, 33(4): 384–5.

Baker, R., Camosso-Stefinovic, J., Gillies, C., Shaw, E.J., Cheater, F., Flottorp, S. and Robertson, N. (2010) Tailored interventions to overcome identified barriers to change: effects on professional practice and health care outcomes. *Cochrane Database of Systematic Reviews*, Issue 3.

Balaskas, J. (1990) *New Active Birth*. London: Thorsons.

Balaskas, J. (1995) *New Active Birth: A Concise Guide to Natural Childbirth*. London: Unwin Paperbacks.

Ball, L., Curtis, P. and Kirkham, M. (2002) *Why Do Midwives Leave?* London: Royal College of Midwives.

Ban Leong, S., Lim Y. and Sia, A. (2008) Early versus late initiation of epidural analgesia for labour. *Cochrane Database of Systematic Reviews*, Issue 3.

Barnett, C., Hundley, V., Cheyne, H. and Kane, F. (2008) 'Not in labour': impact of sending women home in the latent phase. *British Journal of Midwifery*, 16(3): 144–53.

Baskett, T. (2000) A flux of the reds: evolution of active management of the third stage of labour. *Journal of the Royal Society of Medicine*, 93: 489–93.

Beckmann, M.M. and Garrett, A.J. (2006) Antenatal perineal massage for reducing perineal trauma. *Cochrane Database of Systematic Reviews*, Issue 1.

Begley, C. (1990) A comparison of active and physiological management of the third stage of labour. *Midwifery*, 6: 3–17.

Begley, C., Gyte, G., Murphy, D., Devane, D., McDonald, S. and McGuire, W. (2010) Active versus expectant management for women in the third stage of labour. *Cochrane Database of Systematic Reviews*, Issue 7.

bellydancer.org: www.bellydancer.org.uk/bellybab.htm.

Benner, P. (1984) *From Novice to Expert: Excellence and Power in Clinical Nursing Practice*. Menlo Park, CA: Addison-Wesley.

Berg, M. (1997) Problems and promises of the protocol. *Social Science & Medicine*, 44(8): 1081–8.

Bergstrom, L., Richards, L., Proctor, A., Morse, J. and Roberts, J. (2009) Birth talk in second stage labour. *Qualitative Health Research*, 19(7): 954–64.

Bergstrom, L., Richards, L. and Roberts, J. (2010) How caregivers manage pain and distress in second-stage labour. *Journal of Midwifery & Women's Health*, 55(1): 38–45.

Bergstrom, L., Roberts, J., Skillman, L. and Seidel, J. (1992) 'You'll feel me touching you, sweetie': vaginal examinations during the second stage of labour. *Birth*, 19(1): 10–18.

Bergstrom, L., Seedily, J., Schulman-Hull, L. and Roberts, J. (1997) 'I gotta push. Please let me push!': social interactions during the change from first to second stage labour. *Birth*, 24(3): 173–80.

Bergström, M., Kieler, H. and Waldenstrom, U. (2009) Effects of natural childbirth preparation versus standard antenatal education on epidural rates, experience of childbirth and parental stress in mothers and fathers: a randomised controlled multicentre trial. *BJOG*, 116: 1167–76.

Bick, D., MacArthur, C. and Winter, H. (2008) *Postnatal Care: Evidence and Guidelines for Management*, 2nd edn. London: Churchill Livingstone.

Blix, E., Reinar, L. and Klovning, A. and Oian, P. (2005) Prognostic value of the admission test and its effectiveness compared with auscultation only: a systematic review. *BJOG*, 112: 1595–604.

Bloom, S., Casey, B., Schaffer, J., McIntire, D. and Leveno, K. (2006) A randomized trial of coached versus uncoached maternal pushing during the second stage of labor. *American Journal of Obstetrics & Gynecology*, 194: 10–13.

Bloom, S., McIntyre, D., Beimer, M. *et al.* (1998) Lack of effect of walking on labor and delivery. *New England Journal of Medicine*, 339(2): 76–9.

Bloomfield, T. and Gordon, H. (1990) Reaction to blood loss at delivery. *Journal of Obstetrics & Gynaecology*, 10(suppl. 2): S13–S16.

Bo, K., Talseth, T. and Vinsnes, A. (2000) Randomised controlled trial on the effect of pelvic floor muscle training on quality of life and sexual problems in genuine stress incontinent women. *Acta Obstetrica et Gynaecologica Scandinavica*, 79(7): 598–603.

Borup, L., Wurlitzer, W., Hedegaard, U. *et al.* (2009) Acupuncture as pain relief during delivery: a randomised controlled trial. *Birth*, 36(1): 5–12.

Bose, P., Regan, F. and Paterson-Brown, S. (2006) Improving the accuracy of estimated blood loss at obstetric haemorrhage using clinical reconstructions. *BJOG*, 113: 919–24.

Bosomworth, A. and Bettany-Saltikov, J. (2006) Just take a deep breath. *Midirs*, 16(2): 157–65.

Bowen, M. and Selinger, M. (2002) Episiotomy closure comparing enbucrilate tissue adhesive with conventional sutures. *International Journal of Gynecology & Obstetrics*, 78: 201–5.

Boyle, M. (2000) Childbirth in bed: the historical perspective. *The Practising Midwife*, 3(11): 21–4.

Bradley, R. (2008) *Husband Coached Childbirth*. New York: Pergamum.

Bricker, L. and Lavender, T. (2002) Parental opioids for pain relief: a systematic review. *American Journal of Obstetrics & Gynecology*, 186: S94–109.

Browne, J. and Chandra, A. (2009) Slow midwifery. *Women and Birth*, 22: 29–33.

Browning, C. (2000) Using music during childbirth. *Birth*, 27(4): 272–6.

Browning, C. (2001) Music therapy in childbirth: research in practice. *Music Therapy Perceptions*, 19(2): 74–81.

Buchsbaum, G., Chin, M., Glantz, C. and Guzick, D. (2002) Prevalence of urinary incontinence and associated risk factors in a cohort of nuns. *Obstetrics & Gynecology*, 100(2): 226–9.

Buckley, S. (2004) Undisturbed birth: nature's hormonal blueprint for safety, ease and ecstasy. *Midirs*, 14(2): 203–9.

Buckley, S. (2005) *Gentle Birth, Gentle Mothering*. Brisbane: One Moon Press.

Buckley, S. (2010) Sexuality in labour and birth: an intimate perspective. In D. Walsh and S. Downe (eds) *Essential Midwifery Practice: Intrapartum Care*. London: Wiley-Blackwell.

Budd, A. (2000) Acupuncture. In D. Tiran and S. Mack (eds) *Complementary Therapies of Pregnancy and Childbirth*. London: Bailliere Tindall.

Bugg, G., Stanley, E., Bakrt, P., Taggart, M. and Johnston, T. (2006) Outcomes of labours augmented with oxytocin. *European Journal of Obstetrics & Gynecology and Reproductive Biology* 124 (2006) 37–41.

Buhling, K., Schmidt, S., Robinson, J., Klapp, C., Siebert, G. and Dudenhausen, J. (2006) Rate of dyspareunia after delivery in primiparae according to mode of delivery. *European Journal of Obstetrics & Gynecology and Reproductive Biology*, 124: 42–6.

Burns, E., Blamey, C., Ersser, S. *et al.* (2000) The use of aromatherapy in intrapartum midwifery practice: an observational study. *Complementary Therapies in Nursing & Midwifery*, 6: 33–4.

Burns, E., Zobbi, V., Panzeri, D., Oskrochi, R. and Regalia, A. (2007) Aromatherapy in childbirth: a pilot randomised controlled trial. *BJOG*, 114: 838–44.

Burvill, S. (2002) Midwifery diagnosis of labour onset. *British Journal of Midwifery*, 10(10): 600–5.

Byrne, D. and Edmonds, D. (1990) Clinical methods for evaluating progress in first stage of labour. *Lancet*, 335(1681): 122.

Byrom, S., Byrom, A. and Downe, S. (2011) Transformation leadership in midwifery: a nested narrative review. In S. Downe, S. Byrom and L. Simpson (eds) *Essential Midwifery Practice: Leadership, Expertise and Collaborative Working*. London: Wiley-Blackwell.

Byrom, S., Fardella, J., Sandford, J. and Martindale, L. (2010) Collaborating to push boundaries to promote positive birth: an inspirational reflection. *Midirs*, 20(2): 199–205.

Byrom, S., Murray, K. and Thompson, G. (2010) Tales of loss. In D. Walsh and S. Byrom (eds) *Birth Stories for the Soul*. London: Quay Books.

Caldeyro-Barcia, R. (1979) Influence of maternal bearing down efforts during second stage on fetal well-being. *Birth and Family Journal*, 6(1): 7–15.

Caldeyro-Barcia, R., Giussi, G., Storch, E. *et al.* (1979) The influence of maternal bearing down efforts and their effects on fetal heart rate, oxygenation and acid base balance. *Journal of Perinatal Medicine*, 9: 63–7.

Callister, L., Khalaf, I., Semenic, S. *et al.* (2003) The pain of childbirth: perceptions of culturally diverse women. *Pain Management Nursing*, 4(4): 145–54.

Calvert, I. (2000) The evaluation of the use of herbal substances in the bath water of labouring women. Personal communication.

Calvert, I. (2005) Ginger: an essential oil for shortening labour. *The Practising Midwife*, 8(1): 30–4.

Camm, J. (2006) The male midwife: one man's view on childbirth. *Midwives*, 9(6): 224.

Campbell, R. (1997) Place of birth reconsidered. In J. Alexander, V. Levy and C. Roth (eds) *Midwifery Practice: Core Topics 2*. London: Macmillan.

Cardozo, L. and Gleeson, C. (1997) Pregnancy, childbirth and continence. *British Journal of Midwifery*, 5(5): 277–81.

Carlsson, I., Hallberg, L. and Pettersson, K. (2009) Swedish women's experiences of seeking care and being admitted during the latent phase of labour: a grounded theory study. *Midwifery*, 25: 172–80.

Carper, B.A. (1978). Fundamental patterns of knowing in nursing. *Advances in Nursing Science*, 1(1): 13–23.

Carroli, G. and Mignini, L. (2009) Episiotomy for vaginal birth (Cochrane Review). In *The Cochrane Library*, Issue 1. Chichester: John Wiley & Sons, Ltd.

Carroll, D., Tramer, M., McQuay, H., Nye, B. and Moore, A. (1997) Transcutaneous electrical nerve stimulation in labour pain: a systematic review. *British Journal of Obstetrics and Gynaecology*, 104: 169–75.

Carter, S. (2010) Beyond control: body and self in women's childbearing narratives. *Sociology of Health & Illness*, 32(7): 993–1009.

Cepeda, M., Carr, D., Lau, J. and Alvarez, H. (2006) Music for pain relief. *Cochrane Database of Systematic Reveiws*, Issue 2.

Cesario, S. (2004) Re-evaluation of Freidman's labour curve: a pilot study. *Journal of Obstetric, Gynecologic, & Neonatal Nursing*, 33: 713–22.

Chaliha, C., Khullar, V., Stanton, S. *et al.* (2002) Urinary symptoms in pregnancy: are they useful for diagnosis? *British Journal of Obstetrics and Gynaecology*, 109: 1181–3.

Chang, M., Wang, S. and Chen, C. (2002) Effects of massage on pain and anxiety during labour: a randomised controlled trial in Taiwan. *Journal of Advanced Nursing*, 38(1): 68–73.

Chang, S., Chou, M., Lin, L., Lin, Y. and Kuo, S. (2010) Effects of a pushing intervention on pain, fatigue and birthing experiences among Taiwanese women during the second stage of labour. *Midwifery*, doi:10.1016/j.midw.2010.08.009.

Cheng, Y., Hopkins, L., Laros, R., Jr, and Caughey, A. (2007) Duration of the second stage of labor in multiparous women: maternal and neonatal outcomes. *American Journal of Obstetrics & Gynecology*, 196: 585.e1–585.e6.

Cheng, Y., Shaffer, B. and Caughey, A. (2006) The association between persistent occiput posterior position and neonatal outcomes. *Obstetrics & Gynecology*, 107(4): 837–44.

Cheung, N. and Fleming, A. (2011) Case studies of collaboration in the UK and China. In S. Downe, S. Byrom and L. Simpson (eds) *Essential Midwifery Practice: Leadership, Expertise and Collaborative Working*. London: Wiley-Blackwell.

Cheyne, H., Dowding, D. and Hundley, V. (2006) Making the diagnosis of labour: midwives' diagnostic judgement and management decisions. *Journal of Advanced Nursing*, 53(6): 625–35.

Cheyney, M. (2008) Homebirth as systems-challenging praxis: knowledge, power, and intimacy in the birthplace. *Qualitative Health Research*, 18(2): 254–67.

Chuntharapat, S., Petpichetchian, W. and Hatthakit, U. (2008) Yoga during pregnancy: effects on maternal comfort, labour pain and birth outcomes. *Complementary Therapies in Clinical Practice*, 14: 105–15.

Cioffi, J., Swain, J. and Arundell, F. (2010) The decision to suture after childbirth: cues, related factors, knowledge and experience used by midwives. *Midwifery*, 26: 246–55.

Clark, S., Simpson, K., Knox, E. and Garite, T. (2009) Oxytocin: new perspectives on an old drug. *American Journal of Obstetrics & Gynecology*, 35.e1.

Clement, S. (1994) Unwanted vaginal examinations. *British Journal of Midwifery*, 2(8): 368–70.

Clement, S. and Reed, B. (1999) To stitch or not to stitch. *The Practising Midwife*, 2(4): 20–8.

Clinical Negligence Scheme for Trusts (2011) *Maternity Evidence Template: 2011/12 (ET4)*.

Cluett, E.R. and Burns, E. (2009) Immersion in water in labour and birth. *Cochrane Database of Systematic Reviews*, Issue 2.

Cluett, E., Pickering, R. and Getliffe, K. (2004) Randomised controlled trial of labouring in water compared with standard of augmentation for management of dystocia in first stage of labour. *British Medical Journal*, 328: 314.

Coombs, M. and Ersser, S. (2004) Medoca: hegemony in decision-making – a barrier to interdisciplinary working in intensive care? *Journal of Advanced Nursing*, 46(3): 245–52.

Coppen, R. (2005) *Birthing Positions: Do Midwives Know Best?* London: Quay Books.

Coyle, K., Hauck, Y. and Percival, P. (2001a) Normality and collaboration: mothers' perceptions of birth centre versus hospital care. *Midwifery*, 17(3): 182–93.

Coyle, K., Hauck, Y., Percival, P. and Kristjanson, L. (2001b) Ongoing relationships with a personal focus: mother's perceptions of birth centre versus hospital care. *Midwifery*, 17: 171–81.

Crabtree, S. (2008) Midwives constructing 'normal birth'. In S. Downe (ed.) *Normal Childbirth: Evidence and Debate*. London: Elsevier Science.

Cronin, R. and Maude, R. (2010) To suture or not to suture second degree perineal lacerations: what informs this decision? *Midirs*, 20(1): 69–77.

Crowther, S. (2006) Lotus birth: leaving the cord alone. *The Practising Midwife*, 9(6): 12–15.

Cummings, B. and Tiran, D. (2000) Homeopathy for pregnancy and childbirth. In D. Tiran and S. Mack (eds) *Complementary Therapies for Pregnancy and Childbirth*, London: Bailliere Tindall.

Cyna, A., McAuliffe, G. and Andrew, M. (2004) Hypnosis for pain relief in labour and childbirth: a systematic review. *British Journal of Anaesthesia*, 93(4): 505–11.

Dahlen, H. (2010) Undone by fear? Deluded by trust. *Midwifery*, 26: 156–62.

Dahlen, H., Homer, C. and Cooke, M. (2007) Perineal outcomes and maternal comfort related to the application of perineal warm packs in the second stage of labor: a randomized controlled trial. *Birth*, 34(4): 282–90.

Dahlen, H., Homer, C., Leap, N. and Tracy, S. (2010) From social to surgical: historical perspectives on perineal care during labour and birth. *Women and Birth*, doi:1016/j.wombi.2010.09.002.

Dahlen, H., Ryam, M., Homer, C. and Cooke, M. (2007) An Australian prospective cohort study of risk factors for severe perineal truama during childbirth. *Midwifery*, 23: 196–203.

Dandolu, V., Gaughan, J. and Chatwani, A. *et al.* (2005) Risk of recurrence of anal sphincter lacerations. *Obstetrics & Gynecology*, 105: 831–5.

Dannecker, C., Hillemanns, P. and Strauss, A. *et al.* (2004) Episiotomy and perineal tears presumed to be imminent: randomised controlled trial. *Acta Obstetrics et Gynaecologica Scandinavica*, 83: 364–8.

Da Silva, F., de Oliveira, S. and Nobre, M. (2009) A randomised controlled trial evaluating the effect of immersion bath on labour pain. *Midwifery*, 25: 286–94.

Davidson, K., Jacoby, S. and Scott Brown, M. (2000) Prenatal perineal massage: preventing lacerations during delivery. *Journal of Obstetric, Gynecologic, & Neonatal Nursing*, 29(5): 474–9.

Davies, B. (2002) Sources and models for moving research evidence into clinical practice. *Journal of Obstetric, Gynecologic, & Neonatal Nursing*, 31: 558–62.

Davis, B., Johnson, K. and Gaskin, I. (2002) The MANA Curve: describing plateaus in labour using the MANA database. Abstract no. 30, 26th Triennial Congress, ICM, Vienna.

Davis, D. and Walker, K. (2010) Re-discovering the material body in midwifery through an exploration of theories of embodiment. *Midwifery*, 26(4): 457–62.

Davis-Floyd, R. (2003) Home-birth emergencies in the US and Mexico: the trouble with transport. *Social Science & Medicine*, 56: 1911–31.

Davis-Floyd, R. and Davis, E., 1997. Intuition as authoritative knowledge in midwifery and homebirth. In R. Davis-Floyd and C. Sargent (eds) *Childbirth and Authoritative Knowledge*. London: University of California Press, pp. 315–49.

Dawson, P. (2006) Communication between maternity stakeholders. Abstract for New Zealand College of Midwives. Personal communication.

Deave, T., Johnson, D. and Ingram, J. (2008) Transition to parenthood: the needs of parents in pregnancy and early parenthood. *BMC Pregnancy and Childbirth*, 8: 30–41.

Declerq, E., Sakala, C., Corry, M., Applebaum, S. and Risher, P. (2002) *Listening to Mothers: Report of the First National US Survey of Women's Childbearing Experiences*. New York: Maternity Center Association.

Declerq, E., Sakala, C., Corry, M., Applebaum, S. and Risher, P. (2006) Listening to mothers II: report of the Second National U.S. Survey of Women's Childbearing Experiences. *Journal of Perinatal Education*, 16(4): 15–17.

Deering, S., Carlson, N. and Stitely, M. (2004) Perineal body length and lacerations at delivery. *Journal of Reproductive Medicine*, 49(4): 306–10.

Deery, R., Hughes, D. and Kirkham, M. (2010) *Tensions and Barriers in Improving Maternity Care: A Story of a Birth Centre*. Oxford: Radcliffe Publishing.

De Jonge, A. and Lagro-Janssen, A. (2004) Birthing positions: a qualitative study into the views of women about various birthing positions. *Journal of Psychosomatic Obstetrics & Gynecology*, 25: 47–55.

De Jonge, A. and Lagro-Janssen, A. (2007) Increased blood loss in upright birthing positions originates from perineal damage. *BJOG*, 114: 349–55.

De Jonge, A., Teunissen, T. and Lagro-Janssen, A. (2004) Supine position compared to other positions during the second stage of labour: a meta-analytic review. *Journal of Psychosomatic Obstetrics & Gynecology*, 25: 35–45.

De Jonge, A., van de Goes, B., Ravelli, A., Amelink-Verburg, M. and Mol, B. (2009) Perinatal mortality and morbidity in a nationwide cohort of 529 688 low-risk planned home and hospital births. *BJOG*, doi:10.1111/j.1471-0528.2009.02175.x.

De Jonge, A., Teunissen, A., van Diem, M., Scheepers, P. and Lagro-Janssen, A. (2008) Women's positions during the second stage of labour: views of primary care midwives. *Journal of Advanced Nursing*, 63(4): 347–56.

Dencker, A., Berg, M., Bergqvist, L., Ladfors, L., Thorsen, L.S. and Lilja, H. (2009) Early versus delayed oxytocin augmentation in nulliparous women with prolonged labour: a randomised controlled trial. *BJOG*, 116: 530–6.

den Hertog, C., de Groot, A. and van Dongen, P. (2001) History and use of oxytocics. *European Journal of Obstetrics & Gynecology and Reproductive Biology*, 94(1) (suppl.): 8–12.

Denny, M. (1999) Acupuncture in pregnancy. *The Practising Midwife*, 2(4): 29–31.

Department of Health (2008) *High Quality Care for All: NHS Next Stage Review Final Report* [Darzy Report]. London: Department of Health.

de Souza, A., da Costa, C. and Riesco, M. (2006) A comparison of 'hands off' versus 'hands on' techniques for decreasing lacerations during childbirth. *Journal of Midwifery & Women's Health*, 51: 106–11.

Devane, D. (1996) Sexuality and midwifery. *British Journal of Midwifery*, 4(8): 413–20.

Devane, D. and Lalor, J. (2005) Midwives' visual interpretation of intrapartum cardiotocographs: intra- and inter-observer agreement. *Journal of Advanced Nursing*, 52(2): 133–41.

De Vries, R. and Lemmens, T. (2006) The social and cultural shaping of medical evidence: case studies from pharmaceutical research and obstetric science. *Social Science & Medicine*, 62: 2694–706.

D'Gregorio, R. (2010) Obstetric violence: a new legal term introduced in Venezuela. Special editorial. *International Journal of Gynecology & Obstetrics*, 111: 201–2.

Dick-Read, G. (1933) *Natural Childbirth*. London: Heinemann Medical Books.

Dick-Read, G. (1957) *Childbirth without Fear: The Principles and Practice of Natural Childbirth*. London: Heinemann.

Dietz, H. and Schierlitz, L. (2005) Pelvic floor trauma in childbirth: myth or reality? *Australian and New Zealand Journal of Obstetric and Gynaecology*, 45(1): 3–11.

DiMatteo, M., Morton, S., Lepper, H., Damush, T., Carney, M., Pearson, M. and Kahn, K. (1996) Caesarean childbirth and psychosocial outcomes: a meta-analysis. *Health Psychology*, 15(4): 303–14.

DiPiazza, D., Richter, H., Chapman, V., Cliver, S., Neely, C., Chen, C. and Burgio, K. (2006) Risk factors for anal sphincter tear in multiparas. *Obstetrics & Gynecology*, 107(6): 1233–6.

Dixon, L., Fletcher, L., Tracy, S., Guilliland, K., Pairman, S. and Hendry, C. (2009) Midwives' care during the third stage of labour. *New Zealand College of Midwives*, 41: 20–5.

Donnelly, V., Fynes, M. and Campbell, D. (1998) Obstetric events leading to anal sphincter damage. *Obstetrics & Gynecology*, 92: 955–61.

Donnison, J. (1988) *Midwives and Medical Men: A History of the Struggle for the Control of Childbirth*. London: Historical Publications.

Downe, S. (2003) Transition and the second stage of labour. In D. Fraser and A. Cooper (eds) *Myles Textbook for Midwives*, 14th edn. Edinburgh: Churchill Livingstone, pp. 487–505.

Downe, S. and Finlayson, K. (2011) Collaboration: theories, models and maternity care. In S. Downe, S. Byrom and L. Simpson (eds) *Essential Midwifery Practice: Leadership, Expertise and Collaborative Working*. London: Wiley-Blackwell.

Downe, S. and McCourt, C. (2008) From being to becoming: reconstructing childbirth knowledges. In S. Downe (ed.) *Normal Childbirth: Evidence and Debate*, 2nd edn. London: Churchill Livingstone, pp. 3–24.

Downe, S., Gerrett, D. and Renfrew, M. (2004) A prospective randomised controlled trial on the effects of position in the passive second stage of labour on birth outcomes in nulliparous women using epidural analgesia. *Midwifery*, 20(2): 157–68.

Downe, S., Young, C. and Hall Moran, V. (2008) The early pushing urge: practice and discourse. In S. Downe (ed.) *Normal Birth: Evidence and Debate*, 2nd edn. London: Churchill Livingstone.

Downs, F. (1966) Technical innovations: legal implications for nursing. *ANA Clinical Sessions*, 232–7.

Dowswell, T., Bedwell, C., Lavender, T. and Neilson, J.P. (2009) Transcutaneous electrical nerve stimulation (TENS) for pain relief in labour. *Cochrane Database of Systematic Reviews*, Issue 2.

Dudding, T., Vaizey, C. and Camm, M. (2008) Obstetric anal sphincter injury: incidence, risk factors, and management. *Annals of Surgery*, 247(2): 224–37.

Dumoulin, C. and Hay-Smith, J. (2010) Pelvic floor muscle training versus no treatment, or inactive control treatments, for urinary incontinence in women. *Cochrane Database of Systematic Reviews*, Issue 1.

Dunn, P. (1991) Francois Mauriceau (1637–1709) and maternal posture for parturition. *Midirs*, 66: 78–9.

Durham, L. and Collins, M. (1986) The effects of music as a conditioning aid in prepared childbirth education. *Journal of Obstetric, Gynecologic, & Neonatal Nursing*, 15: 268–70.

Durkin, L. (2009) A waterbirth audit. Concurrent session, 3rd International Normal Birth Conference, Grange-over-Sands.

East, C., Begg L. Henshall, N., Marchant, P. and Wallace, K. (2007) Local cooling for relieving pain for perineal pain from perineal trauma sustained during childbirth. *Cochrane Database of Systematic Reviews*, Issue 4.

Eberhard, J., Stein, S. and Geissbuehler, V. (2005) Experience of pain and analgesia with water and land births. *Journal of Psychosomatic Obstetrics & Gynecology*, 26(2): 127–33.

Edwards, N. (2000) Woman planning homebirths: their own views on their relationships with midwives. In M. Kirkham (ed.) *The Midwife–Woman Relationship*, London: Macmillan, pp. 55–91.

Eichenbaum-Pikser, G. and Zasloff, J. (2009) Delayed clamping of the umbilical cord: a review with implication for practice. *Journal of Midwifery & Women's Health*, 54(4): 321–6.

Eid, P., Felisi, E. and Sideri, M. (1993) Applicability of homeopathic caulophyllum thalictroides during labour. *British Homeopathic Journal*, 82(4): 245–8.

Enkin, M. (1992) Commentary: Do I do that? Do I really do that? Like that? *Birth*, 19(1): 19–20.

Enkin, M., Kierse, M., Neilson, J., Crowther, C., Duley, L., Hodnett, E. and Hofmeyr, J. (2000) *A Guide to Effective Care in Pregnancy and Childbirth*. Oxford: Oxford University Press.

Enning Modified APGAR – Scoring for Babies Born in Water (2010). Online: www.mybirthbydesign.com/Enning%20Modified%20APGAR%20Waterbirth.pdf (accessed December 2010).

Eri, T., Blystad, A., Gjengendal, E. and Blaaka, G. (2009) Negotiating credibility: first-time mothers' experiences of contact with the labour ward before hospitalisation. *Midwifery*, doi:10.1016/j.midw.2008.11.005.

Esposito, N.W. (1999) Marginalised women's comparisons of their hospital and free-standing birth centre experience: a contract of inner city birthing centres. *Health Care for Women International*, 20(2): 111–26.

Essex, H. and Pickett, K. (2008) Mothers without companionship during childbirth: an analysis within the millennium cohort study. *Birth*, 35(4): 266–76.

Fahy, K. (1998) Being a midwife or doing midwifery. *Australian College of Midwives Incorporated Journal*, 11(2): 11–16.

Fahy, K. (2009) Third stage of labour care for women at low risk of postpartum haemorrhage. *Journal of Midwifery & Women's Health*, 54: 380–6.

Fahy, K., Foureur, M. and Hastie, C. (2008) *Birth Territory and Midwifery Guardianship*. London: Elsevier.

Fahy, K., Hastie, C., Bisits, A., Marsh, C., Smith, L. and Saxton, A. (2010) Holistic physiological care compared with active management of the third stage of labour for woman at low risk of postpartum haemorrhage: a cohort study. *Women and Birth*, 23: 145–52.

Fannon, M. (2003) Domesticating birth in the hospital: 'family centred' birth and the emergence of 'homelike' birthing rooms. *Antipode*, 35: 513–35.

Farrar, D., Airey, R., Tuffnell, D. and Duley, L. (2009) Care during the third stage of labour: a postal survey of obstetricians and midwives. *Archives of Disease in Childhood. Fetal and Neonatal Edition*, 94 (suppl. 1): Fa40.

Fatherhood Institute (2009) *The Dad Deficit: The Missing Piece in the Maternity Jigsaw*. Online: www.fatherhoodinstitute.org/index.php?id=2&cID=734.

Featherstone, I.E. (1999) Physiological third stage of labour. *British Journal of Midwifery*, 7: 216–21.

Field, T., Hernandez-Reif, M., Taylor, S., Quintino, O. and Burman, I. (1997) Labor pain is reduced by massage therapy. *Journal of Psychosomatic Obstetrics & Gynecology*, 18: 286–91.

Finigan, V. and Davies, S. (2005) 'I just wanted to love him forever': women's lived experience of skin-to-skin contact with their baby immediately after birth. *Evidence Based Midwifery*, 2(2): 59–65.

Finlay, S. and Sandall, J. (2009) 'Someone's rooting for you': Continuity, advocacy and street-level bureaucracy in UK maternal healthcare. *Social Science & Medicine*, 69: 1228–35.

Fleming, V., Hagen, S. and Niven, C. (2003) Does perineal suturing make a difference: the SUNS trial. *British Journal of Obstetrics and Gynaecology*, 110: 684–9.

Flint, C. (1986) *Sensitive Midwifery*. London: Butterworth-Heinemann.

Flint, C. (1993) *Midwifery Teams and Caseloads*. London: Butterworth Heinemann.

Flodgren, G., Parmelli, E., Doumit, G., Gattellari, M., O'Brien, MA, Grimshaw, J. and Eccles, M.P. (2007) Local opinion leaders: effects on professional practice and health care outcomes. *Cochrane Database of Systematic Reviews*, Issue 1.

Flynn, A., Hollins, K. and Lynch, P. (1978) Ambulation in labour. *British Medical Journal*, 2(6137): 591–3.

Fogarty, V. (2008) Intradermal sterile water injections for the relief of lower back pain in labour: a systematic review of the literature. *Women and Birth*, 21: 157–63.

Fontein, J. (2010) The comparison of birth outcomes and birth experiences of low-risk women in different sized midwifery practices in the Netherlands. *Women and Birth*, 23: 103–10.

Forsetlund, L., Bjørndal, A., Rashidian, A., Jamtvedt, G., O'Brien, M.A., Wolf, F., Davis, D., Odgaard-Jensen, J. and Oxman, A.D. (2009) Continuing education meetings and workshops: effects on professional practice and health care outcomes. *Cochrane Database of Systematic Reviews*, Issue 2.

Foster, J. (2005) Innovative practice in birth education. In M. Nolan and J. Foster (eds) *Birth and Parenting Skills: New Directions in Antenatal Education*. London: Elsevier Science.

Foucault, M., 1973. *The Birth of the Clinic: An Archaeology of Medical Perception*. London: Tavistock.

Fraser, W., Marcoux, S., Krauss, I. *et al.* (2000) Multi-centre, randomized controlled trial of delayed pushing for nulliparous women in the second stage of labor with continuous epidural analgesia. *American Journal of Obstetrics & Gynecology*, 182: 1165–72.

Freeman, R., Macaulay, A. and Chamberlain, G. (1986) Randomised controlled trial of self-hypnosis for analgesia in labour. *British Medical Journal*, 292: 657–8.

Frenea, S., Chirossel, C., Rodriguez, R. and Baguet, J.P. (2004) The effects of prolonged ambulation on labour with epidural analgesia. *Obstetric Anesthesia*, 98: 224–9.

Friedman, E. (1954) The graphic analysis of labor. *American Journal of Obstetrics & Gynecology*, 68: 1568–75.

Friedman, E. (1955) Primigravid labor: a graphicostatistical analysis. *Obstetrics & Gynecology*, 6: 567–89.

Frigoletto, F., Lieberman, E. and Lang, J. (1995) A clinical trial active management of labor. *New England Journal of Medicine*, 333: 745–50.

Fry, J. (2007a) Are there other ways of knowing? An exploration of intuition as a source of authoritative knowledge in childbirth. *Midirs* 17(3): 325–8.

Fry, J. (2007b) Physiological third stage of labour: support it or lose it. *British Journal of Midwifery*, 15: 693–5.

Frye, A. (2004) *Holistic Midwifery Volume II: Care of the Mother and Baby from Onset of Labour through the First Hours after Birth*. Portland: Labry's Press.

Fullerton, J., Navarro, A. and Young, H. (2007) Outcomes of planned home birth: an integrative review. *Journal of Midwifery & Women's Health*, 52: 323–33.

Gabbay, J. and le May, A. (2004) Evidence based guidelines or collectively constructed 'mindlines?' Ethnographic study of knowledge management in primary care. *British Medical Journal*, 329: 1–5.

Gagnon, A.J. and Sandall, J. (2007) Individual or group antenatal education for childbirth or parenthood, or both. *Cochrane Database of Systematic Reviews*, Issue 3.

Gagnon, A., Meier, K. and Waghom, K. (2007) Continuity of nursing care and its link to caesarean birth rate. *Birth*, 34(1): 26–32.

Gardberg, M. and Tuppurainen, M. (1994) Anterior placental location predisposes for occiput posterior presentation near term. *Acta Obstetrica et Gynaecologica*, 73: 151–2.

Garland, D. (2010) *Revisiting Waterbirth: An Attitude to Care*. London: Palgrave Macmillan.

Gaskin, I. (2002) The frequency of reported orgasms in labour and birth in a population of unmedicated women. Abstract no. 310, 26th Triennial Congress, ICM, Vienna.

Gaskin, I.M. (2003) Going backwards: the concept of 'pasmo'. *The Practising Midwife* 6(8): 34–6.

Gaskin, I.M. (2004) Understanding birth and sphincter law. *British Journal of Midwifery*, 12(9): 540, 542.

Geissbuehler, V., Stein, S. and Eberhard, J. (2004) Waterbirth compared with landbirths: an observational study of nine years. *Journal of Perinatal Medicine* 32(4): 308–14.

Gemynthe, A., Langhoff-Ross, J., Sahl, S. and Knudsen, J. (1996) New VICRYL formulation: an improved method of perineal repair? *British Journal of Midwifery*, 4(5): 230–4.

Gerdin, E., Sverrisdottir, G., Badi, A., Carlsson, B. and Graf, W. (2007) The role of maternal age and episiotomy in the risk of anal sphincter tears during childbirth. *Australian and New Zealand Journal of Obstetrics and Gynaecology*, 47(4): 286–90.

Gjerris, A., Staer-Jensen, J., Jorgensen, J. *et al.* (2008) Umbilical cord blood lactate: a valuable tool in the assessment of fetal metabolic acidosis. *European Journal of Obstetrics & Gynecology and Reproductive Biology*, 139: 16–20.

Glazener, C., Herbison, G., Wilson, P. *et al.* (2001) Conservative management of persistent postnatal urinary and faecal incontinence: randomised controlled trial. *British Medical Journal*, 323: 593.

Goer, H. (2010) Cruelty in maternity wards: fifty years later. *Journal of Perinatal Education*, 19(3): 33–42.

Golara, M., Plaat, F. and Shennan, A. (2002) Upright versus recumbent position in the second stage of labour in women with combined spinal-epidural analgesia. *International Journal of Obstetric Anaesthesia*, 11: 19–22.

Gordon, B. (1998) The Ipswich Childbirth Study: 1. A randomised evaluation of 2-stage post-partum perineal repair leaving the skin unsutured. *British Journal of Obstetrics and Gynaecology*, 105(4): 435–40.

Gottvall, K., Allebeck, P. and Ekeus, C. (2007) Risk factors for anal sphincter tears: the importance of maternal position. *BJOG*, 114(10): 1266–72.

Gould, D. (2000) Normal labour: a concept analysis. *Journal of Advanced Nursing*, 31(2): 418–27.

Graham, E., Ruis, K. and Hartman, A. (2008) A systematic review of the role of intrapartum hypoxia-ischemia in the causation of neonatal encephalopathy. *American Journal of Obstetrics & Gynecology*, December: 587–95.

Graham, I. (1997) *Episiotomy: Challenging Obstetric Interventions*. London: Blackwell.

Greatbatch, D., Hanlon, G., Goode, J., O'Caithain, A.O., Strangleman, T. and Luff, D. (2005) Telephone triage, expert systems and clinical expertise. *Sociology of Health & Illness*, 27(6): 802–30.

Green, J. (1999) Commentary: what is this thing called 'control'? *Birth*, 26(1): 51.

Green, J. and Baston, H. (2007) Have women become more willing to accept obstetric interventions and does this relate to mode of birth? Data from a prospective study. *Birth*, 34: 1–8.

Green, J.M., Coupland, V.A. and Kitzinger, J. (1998) *Great Expectations: A Prospective Study of Women's Expectations and Experiences of Childbirth*. London: Butterworth-Heinemann.

Greene, R., Gardeil, F. and Turner, M. (1997) Long-term implications of caesarean section. *American Journal of Obstetrics & Gynecology*, 176(1): 254–5.

Greer, J. (2010) Are midwives irrational or afraid? *Evidence Based Midwifery*, 8(2): 47–52.

Grol, R. (1997) Personal paper: beliefs and evidence in changing clinical practice. *British Medical Journal*, 315: 418–21.

Grol, R. and Grimshaw, J. (2003) From best evidence to best practice: effective implementation of change in patient's care. *Lancet*, 362: 1225–30.

Gross, M., Haunschild, T., Stoexen, T., Methner, V. and Guenter, H. (2003) Women's recognition of the spontaneous onset of labour. *Birth*, 30(4): 267–71.

Gross, M., Hecker, H., Matterne, A., Guenter, H. and Keirse, M. (2006) Does the way that women experience the onset of labour influence the duration of labour? *BJOG*, 113: 289–94.

Gulmezoglu, A., Forna, F., Villar, J. and Hofmeyr, G. (2006) Prostaglandins for prevention for postpartum haemorrhage. *Cochrane Database of Systematic Reviews*, Issue 3.

Gupta, J.K. and Hofmeyr, G.J. (2006) Position for women during second stage of labour (Cochrane Review). In *The Cochrane Library*, Issue 4. Chichester: John Wiley & Sons, Ltd.

Gupta, J.K., Hofmeyr, G.J. and Smyth, R.M.D. (2004) Position in the second stage of labour for women without epidural anaesthesia. *Cochrane Database of Systematic Reviews*, Issue 1.

Gurewitsch, E., Diament, P., Fong, J., Huang, G.H., Popovtzer, A., Weinstein, D. and Chervenak, F.A. (2002) The labor curve of the grand multipara: Does progress of labor continue to improve with additional childbearing? *American Journal of Obstetrics & Gynecology*, 186: 1331–8.

Gyte, G. (1994) Evaluation of the meta-analyses on the effects on both mother and baby, of the various components of 'active' management of the third stage of labour. *Midwifery*, 10: 183–99.

Gyte, G., Dodwell, M., Newburn, M., Sandall, J., MacFarlane, A. and Bewley, S. (2010) Findings of meta-analysis cannot be relied on. *British Journal of Medicine*, 341: c4033.

Haggerty, J., Reid, R., Freeman, G., Starfield, B., Adair, C. and McKendry, R. (2005) Continuity of care: a multidisciplinary review. *British Medical Journal*, 327: 1219–21.

Hall, J. (2001) *Midwifery Mind and Spirit*. Oxford: Books for Midwives Press.

Hall, S. and Holloway, I. (1998) Staying in control: women's experience of labour in water. *Midwifery*, 14(1): 30–6.

Hally McCrea, B., Wright, M. and Murphy-Black, T. (1998) Differences in midwives' approaches to pain relief in labour. *Midwifery*, 14(3): 174–80.

Handa, V., Danielsen, B. and Gilbert, W. (2001) Obstetric anal sphincter lacerations. *Obstetrics & Gynecology*, 98: 225–30.

Handa, V., Harris, T. and Ostergard, D. (1996) Protecting the pelvic floor: obstetric management to prevent incontinence and pelvic organ collapse. *Obstetrics & Gynecology*, 88: 470–8.

Hannah, M., Hannah, J., Hewson, S., Hodnett, E., Saigal, S., Willan, A. and Term Breech Trial Collaborative (2000) Planned caesarean section versus planned vaginal birth for breech presentation at term: a randomised multi-centre trial. *The Lancet*, 356(9239): 1375–83.

Hannestad, Y.S., Rortveit, G., Dalveit, A.K. and Hunskaar, S. (2003) Are smoking and other lifestyle factors associated with female urinary incontinence? The Norwegian EPINCONT study. *British Journal of Obstetrics and Gynaecology*, 110: 247–54.

Hansen, S., Clark, S. and Foster, J. (2002) Active pushing versus passive fetal descent in the second stage of labour: a randomised controlled trial. *Obstetrics & Gynecology*, 99: 29–34.

Hantoushzadeh, S., Alhusseini, N. and Lebasch, A. (2007) The effects of acupuncture during labour on nulliparous women: a randomised controlled trial. *Australian and New Zealand Journal of Obstetrics and Gynaecology*, 47: 26–30.

Harmon, T., Hynan, M. and Tyre, T. (1990) Improved obstetric outcomes using hypnotic analgesia and skill mastery combined with childbirth education. *Journal of Consulting and Clinical Psychology*, 58(5): 525–30.

Harris, T. (2001) Changing the focus for the third stage of labour. *British Journal of Midwifery*, 9(1): 7–12.

Harrison, J. (1999) Fetal perspectives on labour. *British Journal of Midwifery*, 7(10): 643–7.

Hastie, C. and Fahy, K. (2009) Optimising psychophysiology in the third stage of labour: theory applied to practice. *Women and Birth*, 22: 89–96.

Hatem, M., Sandall, J., Devane, D., Soltani, H. and Gates, S. (2008) Midwife-led versus other models of care for childbearing women. *Cochrane Database of Systematic Reviews*, Issue 4.

Hauck, Y., Rivers, C. and Doherty, K. (2008) Women's experiences of using a Snoezelen room during labour in Western Australia. *Midwifery*, 24: 460–70.

Haverkamp, A., Thompson, H., McFee, J. *et al.* (1976) The evaluation of continuous fetal heart rate monitoring in high-risk pregnancy. *American Journal of Obstetrics & Gynecology*, 125(3): 310–20.

Hay-Smith, J., Mørkved, S., Fairbrother, K.A. and Herbison, G.P. (2008) Pelvic floor muscle training for prevention and treatment of urinary and faecal incontinence in antenatal and postnatal women. *Cochrane Database of Systematic Reviews*, Issue 4.

Head, M. (1993) Dropping stitches. *Nursing Times*, 89(33): 64–5.

Healthcare Commission (2007; 10 January 2010). Women's experiences of maternity care in the NHS in England: key findings from a survey of NHS trusts carried out in 2007. Online: www.birthchoiceuk.com/BirthChoiceUKFrame.htm?www.birthchoiceuk.com/HealthCare-CommissionSurvey/Q220.htm.

Hedayati, H., Parsons, J. and Crowther, C.A. (2005) Topically applied anaesthetics for treating perineal pain after childbirth. *Cochrane Database of Systematic Reviews*, Issue 2.

Hedayati, H., Parsons, J. and Crowther, C.A. (2009) Rectal analgesia for pain from perineal trauma following childbirth (Cochrane Review). In *The Cochrane Library*, Issue 4. Chichester: John Wiley & Sons, Ltd.

Heelbeck, L. (1999) Administration of pethidine in labour. *British Journal of Midwifery*, 7(6): 372–7.

Heinze, S. and Sleigh, M. (2003) Epidural or no epidural anaesthesia: relationships between beliefs about childbirth and pain control choices. *Journal of Reproductive and Infant Psychology*, 21(4): 323–34.

Hemminki, E. (1996) Impact of caesarean section on future pregnancy: a review of cohort studies. *Paediatric and Perinatal Epidemiology*, 10(4): 366–79.

Hemminki, E. and Saarikoski, S. (1983) Ambulation and delayed amniotomy in the first stage of labour. *European Journal of Obstetrics & Gynecology and Reproductive Biology*, 15: 129–39.

Henderson, J., Dickenson, J., Evans, S. *et al.* (2003) Impact of intrapartum analgesia on breastfeeding duration. *Australian and New Zealand Journal of Obstetrics and Gynaecology*, 43(5): 372.

Henley-Einion, A. (2007) The ectasy of the spirit: five rhythms of healing. *The Practising Midwife*, 10(3): 20–3.

Herbst, A. and Ingemarsson, I. (1994) Intermittent versus continuous electronic fetal monitoring in labour: a randomised study. *British Journal of Obstetrics and Gynaecology*, 101: 663–8.

Hillan, E. (1991) Electronic fetal monitoring: more problems than benefits? *Midirs*, 1(3): 249–51.

Hindley, C., Hinsliff, S. and Thomson, A. (2005) Developing a tool to appraise fetal monitoring guidelines for women at low obstetric risk. *Journal of Advanced Nursing*, 52(3): 307–14.

Hindley, C., Hinsliff, S. and Thomson, A. (2006) English midwives' views and experiences of intrapartum fetal heart rate monitoring in women at low obstetric risk: conflicts and compromises. *Journal of Midwifery & Women's Health*, 51(5): 354–60.

Hinova, A. and Fernando, R. (2009) Systemic remifentanil for labor analgesia. *Anaethesia and Analgesia*, 109(6): 1925–9.

Hinshaw, K., Simpson, S., Cummings, S., Hildreth, A. and Thorton, J. (2008) A randomised controlled trial of early versus delayed oxytocin augmentation to treat primary dysfunctional labour in nulliparous women. *BJOG*, 115: 1289–96.

Hjelmstedt, A., Shenoy, S., Steiner-Victorin, E. and Lekander, M. (2010) Acupressure to reduce labour pain: a randomised controlled trial. *Acta Obstetrica et Gynecologica*, 89: 1453–9.

Hobbs, L. (1998) Assessing cervical dilatation without VEs. *The Practising Midwife*, 1(11): 34–5.

Hodnett, E. (2002) Pain and women's satisfaction with the experience of childbirth: a systematic review. *American Journal of Obstetrics & Gynecology*, 186: S160–72.

Hodnett, E., Stremler, R., Willan, A. *et al.* (2008) Effects on birth outcomes of a formalised approach to care in hospital labour assessments units: international, randomised controlled trial. *British Medical Journal*, 337(a1021): 1–8.

Hodnett, E., Stremler, R., Westion, J. and McKeever, P. (2009) Re-conceptualising the hospital labour room: the PLACE (Pregnant and labouring in an ambient clinical environment) pilot trial. *Birth*, 36(2): 159–66.

Hodnett, E.D. (2008) Continuity of caregivers for care during pregnancy and childbirth (Cochrane Review). In *The Cochrane Library*, Issue 2. Chichester: John Wiley & Sons, Ltd.

Hodnett, E.D., Downe, S., Walsh, D. and Weston, J. (2010) Alternative versus conventional institutional settings for birth. *Cochrane Database of Systematic Reviews*, Issue 3.

Hodnett, E.D., Gates, S., Hofmeyr, G.J. and Sakala, C. (2009) Continuous support for women during childbirth (Cochrane Review). In *The Cochrane Library*, Issue 1. Chichester: John Wiley & Sons, Ltd.

Hodnett, E.D., Gates, S., Hofmeyr, G.J., Sakala, C. and Weston, J. (2011) Continuous support for women during childbirth. *Cochrane Database of Systematic Reviews*, Issue 2.

Hofmeyr, G.J. and Kulier, R. (2009) Hands/knees posture in late pregnancy or labour for fetal malposition (lateral or posterior) (Cochrane Review). In *The Cochrane Library*, Issue 1. Chichester: John Wiley & Sons, Ltd.

Homer, C., Davis, G., Brodie, P. *et al.* (2001) Collaboration in maternity care: a randomised trial comparing community-based continuity of care with standard hospital care. *British Journal of Obstetrics and Gynaecology*, 108: 16–22.

Hundley, V. (2000) Raising research awareness among midwives and nurses: does it work? *Journal of Advanced Nursing*, 31(1): 78–86.

Hunt, S. and Symonds, A. (1995) *The Social Meaning of Midwifery*. Basingstoke: Macmillan.

Hunter, B. and Deery, R. (2009) *Managing Emotions in Midwifery and Reproductive Health Care*. London: Palgrave Press.

Hunter, B. and Segrott, J. (2008) Re-mapping client journeys and professional identities: a review of the literature on clinical pathways. *International Journal of Nursing Studies*, 45: 608–25.

Hunter, S., Hofmeyr, G. and Kulier, R. (2007) Hands and knees posture in late pregnancy or labour for fetal malposition (lateral or posterior). *Cochrane Database of Systematic Reviews*, Issue 4.

Hutton, E. and Hassan, E. (2007) Late versus early clamping of the umbilical cord in full-term neonates: systematic review and meta-analysis of controlled trials. *Journal of the American Medical Association*, 297: 1241–52.

Hutton, E., Kasperink, M., Rutten, M., Reitsma, A. and Wainman, B. (2009) Sterile water injection for labour pain: a systematic review and meta-analysis of randomised controlled trials. *BJOG*, 116: 1158–66.

Ickovics, J., Trace, S., Kershaw, C. and Westdahl, U. (2007) Group prenatal care and perinatal outcomes: a randomized controlled trial. *Obstetrics & Gynecology*, 110(2) (pt 1): 330–9.

Imseis, H., Trout, W. and Gabbe, S. (1999) The microbiologic effect of digital cervical examination. *American Journal of Obstetrics & Gynecology*, 180(3): 578–80.

Inch, S. (1985) Management of the third stage of labour, another cascade of intervention. *Midwifery*, 1(2): 114–22.

Inch, S. (1988) Physiology of third stage of labour. *Midwives Chronicle and Nursing Notes*, 101: 42–3.

ISIS Birth Centre (2007) Audit data of physiological birth practice 2005–6. Personal communication.

Jackson, D., Lang, J., Ecker, J., Swartz, W. and Heeren, T. (2003a) Impact of collaborative management and early labour admission in labour on method of delivery. *Journal of Obstetric, Gynecologic, & Neonatal Nursing*, 32(2): 147–57.

Jackson, D., Lang, J., Swartz, W. *et al.* (2003b) Outcomes, safety and resource utilization in a collaborative care birth centre program compared with traditional physician-based perinatal care. *American Journal of Public Health*, 93: 999–1006.

Jacobson, B., Nyberg, K., Eklund, G. *et al.* (1988) Obstetric pain medication and eventual adult amphetamine addiction in offspring. *Acta Obstetrics et Gynaecologica Scandinavica*, 67(8): 677–82.

Jacobson, B., Nyberg, K., Gronbladh, L. *et al.* (1990) Opiate addiction in adult offspring through possible imprinting after obstetric treatment. *British Medical Journal*, 301(6760): 1067–70.

Jamtvedt, G., Young, J.M., Kristofferson, D.T., Thomson O'Brien, M.A. and Oxman, A.D. (2006) Audit and feedback: effects on professional practice and health care outcomes (Cochrane Review). In *The Cochrane Library*, Issue 3. Chichester: John Wiley & Sons, Ltd.

Janni, W., Schiessl, B., Peschers, U. *et al.* (2002) The prognostic impact of a prolonged second stage of labour on maternal and fetal outcome. *Acta Obstetrica Gynaecologica Scandinavia*, 81: 214–21.

Janssen, P.A., Iker, C.E. and Carty, E.A. (2003) Early labour assessment and support at home: a randomized controlled trial. *Journal of Gynaecology Canada*, 25: 734–41.

Janssen, P., Saxell, L., Page, L. and Klein, M. (2009) Outcomes of planned home birth with registered midwife versus hospital birth with midwife or physician. *Canadian Medical Association Journal*, 181(6–7): 377–83.

Janssen, P., Still, D., Klein, M., Singer, J. *et al.* (2006) Early labor assessment and support at home versus telephone triage. *Obstetrics & Gynecology*, 108(6): 1463–9.

Jarcho, J. (1934) *Postures and Practices during Labour among Primitive Peoples*. New York: Paul Hoeber.

Jefford, E., Fahy, K. and Sundin, D. (2010) A review of the literature: midwifery decision-making and birth. *Women and Birth*, 23: 127–34.

Johns, C. (1995) The value of reflective practice in nursing. *Journal of Clinical Nursing*, 4(1): 23–30.

Johnson, P. (1996) Birth under water: to breathe or not to breathe. *British Journal of Obstetrics and Gynaecology*, 103: 202–8.

Johnston, J. (2004) The nesting instinct. *Birth Matters Journal*, 8(2): 21–2.

Johnstone, F., Aboelmagd, M. and Harouny, A. (1987) Maternal position in the second stage of labour and fetal acid base status. *British Journal of Obstetrics and Gynaecology*, 94(8): 753–7.

Jonsson, M., Norder-Linderberg, S., Ostlund, I. and Hanson, U. (2008) Acidemia at birth, related to obstetric characteristics and to oxytocin use during the last two hours of labour. *Acta Obstetrica Gynaecological Scandinavia*, 87: 745–50.

Jordan, S., Emery, S., Bradshaw, C. *et al.* (2005) The impact of intrapartum analgesia on infant feeding. *British Journal of Obstetrics and Gynaecology*, 112(7): 927–30.

Jouppila, R., Jouppila, P. and Karlqvist, K. (1983) Maternal and umbilical venous plasma immunoreactive beta-endorphin levels during labor with and without epidural analgesia. *American Journal of Obstetrics & Gynecology*, 147(7): 799–802.

justbewell.com: www.justbewell.com/aboutus/nlp_neuro_linguistic_programming_london.html.

Kainz, G., Eliasson, M. and von Post, I. (2010) The child's father, an important person for the mother's well-being during the childbirth: a hermeneutic study. *Health Care for Women International*, 31(7): 621–35.

Kariminia, A., Chamberlain, M., Keogh, J. and Shea, A. (2004) Randomised controlled trial of effects of hands and knees posturing on incidence of occipito posterior position at birth. *British Medical Journal*, 328: 490.

Kavanagh, J., Kelly, A.J. and Thomas, J. (2009a) Breast stimulation for cervical ripening and induction of labour (Cochrane Review). In *The Cochrane Library*, Issue 1. Chichester, UK: John Wiley & Sons, Ltd.

Kavanagh, J., Kelly, A.J. and Thomas, J. (2009b) Sexual intercourse for cervical ripening and induction of labour (Cochrane Review). In *The Cochrane Library*, Issue 1. Chichester, UK: John Wiley & Sons, Ltd.

Kemp, J. and Sandall, J. (2008) Normal birth, magical birth: the role of the 36-week birth talk in caseload midwifery practice. *Midwifery*: doi:10.1016/j.midw.2008.07.002.

Kennedy, H. (2000) A model of exemplary midwifery practice: results of a Delphi study including commentary by K. Ernst. *Journal of Midwifery & Women's Health*, 45 (1): 4–19.

Kennedy, H., Leap, N. and Anderson, T. (2010) Midwifery presence: philosophy, science, and art. In D. Walsh and S. Downe (eds) *Essential Skills for Intrapartum Care*. London: Wiley-Blackwell.

Kennedy, H., Shannon, M., Chuahorm, U. and Kravetz, M. (2004) The landscape of caring for women: a narrative study of midwifery practice. *Journal of Midwifery & Women's Health*, 49: 14–23.

Kesselheim, A. and Studdert, D. (2006) Characteristics of physicians who frequently act as expert witnesses in neurological birth injury litigation. *Obstetrics & Gynecology*, 108(2): 273–9.

Kettle, C., Dowswell, T. and Ismail, K. (2010) Absorbable suture material for primary repair of episiotomy and second degree tears. *Cochrane Database of Systematic Reviews*, Issue 6.

Kettle, C., Hills, R. and Ismail, K. (2007) Continuous versus interrupted sutures for repair of episiotomy or second degree tears. *Cochrane Database of Systematic Reviews*, Issue 4.

Kettle, C., Hills, R., Jones, P., Darby, L., Gray, R. and Johanson, R. (2002) Continuous versus interrupted perineal repair with standard or rapidly absorbed sutures after spontaneous vaginal birth: a randomised controlled trial. *The Lancet*, 359: 2217–23.

Khoda Karami, N., Safarzadeh, A. and Fathizadeh, N. (2007) Effect of massage therapy on severity of pain and outcomes of labour in primipara. *Iranian Journal of Nursing and Midwifery Research*, 12(1): 6.

Kirkham, M. (1989) Midwives and information-giving during labour. In S. Robinson and A. Thomson (eds) *Midwives, Research and Childbirth, Volume 1*, London: Chapman & Hall.

Kirkham, M. (1995) Using personal planning to meet the challenge of changing childbirth. In *The Challenge of Changing Childbirth: Midwifery Educational Resource Pack*, Section 1. London: ENB.

Kirkham, M. (1999) The culture of midwifery in the National Health Service in England. *Journal of Advanced Nursing*, 30: 732–9.

Kirkham, M. (2004) *Informed Choice in Maternity Care*. London: Palgrave Macmillan.

Kirkham, M. (2005) Trapped by thinking opposites. Keynote Address, International Congress of Midwives, Brisbane.

Kirkham, M. (2010) *The Midwife–Mother Relationship*, 2nd edn. Oxford: Palgrave Macmillan.

Kirkham, M., Stapleton, H., Thomas, G. and Curtis, P. (2000) Checking not listening: how midwives cope. *British Journal of Midwifery*, 10(7): 447–50.

Kirkman, S. (2000) The midwife and pelvic floor dysfunction. *The Practising Midwife*, 3(8): 20–2.

Kitzinger, J. (1990) Strategies of the early childbirth movement: a case study of the national childbirth trust. In J. Garcia, R. Kilpatrick and M. Richards (eds) *The Politics of Maternity Care*. London: Clarendon Paperbacks.

Kitzinger, S. (1977) *Education and Counselling for Childbirth*. London: Bailliere Tindall.

Kitzinger, S. (2000) *Rediscovering Birth*. London: Little Brown and Company.

Kitzinger, S. (2002) *Birth Your Way: Choosing Birth at Home or in a Birth Centre*. London: Dorling Kindersley.

Kitzinger, S. (2004) *The New Experience of Childbirth*. London: Orion.

Kitzinger, S. (2005) *The Politics of Birth*. London: Elsevier.

Kjaergaard, H., Foldgast, A. and Dykes, A. (2007) Experiences of non-progressive and augmented labour among nulliparous women: a qualitative interview study in a grounded theory approach. *BMC Pregnancy and Childbirth*, 7: 15.

Kjærgaard, H., Olsen, J. and Ottesen, B. (2008) Obstetric risk indicators for labour dystocia in nulliparous women: a multi-centre cohort study. *BMC Pregnancy and Childbirth*: doi:10.1186/1471-2393-8-45.

Klassen, P. (1998) Sliding around between pain and pleasure: Home birth and visionary pain. *Scottish Journal of Religious Studies*, 19(1): 45–67.

Klein, M. (2006) In the literature: epidural analgesia – does it or doesn't it? *Birth*, 33(1): 74–6.

Knauth, D. and Haloburdo, E. (1986) Effects of pushing techniques in birthing chair on length of second stage of labour. *Nursing Research*, 35: 49–51.

Krehbiel, D., Poindron, P. and Levy, F. (1987) Peridural anaesthesia disturbs maternal behaviour in primiparous and multiparous parturient ewes. *Physiological Behaviour*, 40(4): 463–72.

Kulier, R., Gee, H. and Khan, K. (2008) Five steps from evidence to effect: exercising clinical freedom to implement research findings. *BJOG*, 115: 1197–202.

Kyeong Lee, M., Bok Chang, S. and Kang, D. (2004) Effects of SP6 acupressure on labour pain and length of delivery time in women during labour. *Journal of Alternative and Complementary Medicine*, 10(6): 959–65.

Labrecque, M., Eason, E., Marcoux, S. *et al.* (1999) Randomised controlled trial of prevention of perineal trauma by perineal massage during pregnancy. *American Journal of Obstetrics & Gynecology*, 180: 593–600.

Laine, K., Pirhonen, T., Rolland, R. and Pirhonen, J. (2008) Decreasing the incidence of anal sphincter tears during delivery. *Obstetrics & Gynecology*, 111(5): 1053–7.

Lal, M., Mann, C., Callender, R. and Radley, S. (2003) Does caesarean delivery prevent anal incontinence? *Obstetrics & Gynecology*, 101: 305–12.

Lang, A., Sorrell, J., Rodgers, S. and Lebeck, M. (2006) Anxiety sensitivity as a predictor of labor pain. *European Journal of Pain*, 10: 263–70.

Langley, V., Thoburn, A., Shaw, S. and Barton, A. (2006) Second degree tears: to suture or not? A randomised controlled trial. *British Journal of Midwifery*, 14(9): 550–4.

Lankshear, G., Ettorre, E. and Mason, D. (2005) Decision-making, uncertainty and risk: Exploring the complexity of work processes in NHS delivery suites. *Health, Risk & Society*, 7(4): 361–77.

Lauritzen, S. and Sachs, L. (2001) Normality, risk and the future: implicit communication of threat in health surveillance. *Sociology of Health & Illness*, 23(4): 497–516.

Laursen, M., Hedegaard, M., Johansen, C. and Danish National Birth Cohort (2008) Fear of childbirth and temporal changes among nulliparous women in the Danish National Birth Cohort. *BJOG*, 115: 354–6.

Laursen, M., Johansen, C. and Hedegaard, M. (2009) Fear of childbirth and risk for birth complications in nulliparous women in the Danish National Birth Cohort. *BJOG*, 116: 1350–5.

Lauzon, L. and Hodnett, E. (2001) Labour assessment programs to delay admission to labour wards. *Cochrane Database of Systematic Reviews*, Issue 3.

Lavender, T. and Chapple, J. (2004) An exploration of midwives' views of the current system of maternity care in England. *Midwifery*, 20(4): 324–34.

Lavender, T., Alfirevic, Z. and Walkinshaw, S. (2006) Effects of different partogram action lines on birth outcomes: a randomised controlled trial. *Obstetrics & Gynecology*, 108(2): 295–302.

Lavender, T., Hart, A. and Smyth, R. (2008) Effects of partogram use on outcomes for women in spontaneous labour at term. *Cochrane Database of Systematic Reviews*, Issue 4.

Lavin, J. and McGregor, J. (1992) Native American childbirth on the western plains. *International Journal of Feto-Maternal Medicine*, 5(3): 125–33.

Lawrence, A., Lewis, L., Hofmeyr, J. *et al.* (2009) Maternal positions and mobility during first stage of labour. *Cochrane Systematic Reviews*, Issue 4.

Laws, P., Tracy, S. and Sullivan, E. (2010) Perinatal outcomes of women intending to give birth in birth centers in Australia. *Birth*, 37(1): 28–36.

Leap, N. (2000a) Pain in labour towards a midwifery perspective. *Midirs Midwifery Digest*, 10(1): 49–53.

Leap, N. (2000b). The less we do, the more we give. In M. Kirkham (ed.) *The Midwife–Mother Relationship*. New York: Palgrave Macmillan, pp. 1–17.

Leap, N. (2010) Working with pain in labour: an overview of evidence. *New Digest*, 49: 22–6.

Leap, N. and Anderson, P. (2008) The role of pain in normal birth and the empowerment of women. In S. Downe (ed.) *Normal Childbirth: Evidence and Debate*, 2nd edn. London: Churchill Livingstone, pp. 25–40.

Leap, N., Sandall, J., Buckland, S. and Huber, U. (2010) Journey to confidence: women's experiences of pain in labour and relational continuity of care. *Journal of Midwifery & Women's Health*, 55: 234–42.

Leboyer, F. (2002) *Birth without Violence*. London: 1st Healing Arts Press.

Lee, B. (2004) Normal birth: is it possible in the 21st century? *Midwives*, 7(9): 396–7.

Leeman, L., Rogers, R., Greulich, B. and Albers, L. (2007) Do unsutured second-degree lacerations affect postpartum functional outcomes? *Journal of American Board of Family Medicine*, 20: 451–7.

Lepori, B., Foureur, M. and Hastie, C. (2008) The moving, feeling and dreaming body guides architectural design. In K. Fahy, M. Foureur and C. Hastie (eds) *Birth Territory and Midwifery Guardianship*. London: Elsevier.

Levy, V. (1999) Maintaining equilibrium: a grounded theory study of the processes involved when women make informed choices during pregnancy. *Midwifery*, 15: 109–19.

Lewin, K. (1951) *Field Theory in Social Science*. New York: Harper & Row.

Lieberman, E. and O'Donoghue, C. (2002) Unintended effects of epidural analgesia during labor. *American Journal of Obstetrics & Gynecology*, 186: S31–68.

Lieberman, E., Davidson, K., Lee-Parritz, A. and Shearer, E. (2005) Changes in fetal position during labor and their association with epidural analgesia. *Obstetrics & Gynecology*, 105(5): 974–82.

Liisberg, G. (1989) Easier births using reflexology. *Tidsskrift for Jordemodre*, 3.

Lindgren, H., Brink, A. and Klinberg-Allvin, M. (2011) Fear causes tears: perineal injuries in home birth settings – a Swedish interview study. *BMC Pregnancy and Childbirth*, 11(6): 1–8.

Lindgren, H., Hildingsson, I. and Christensson, K. (2008a) Outcomes of planned homebirth compared to hospital birth in Sweden between 1992 and 2004: a population-based register study. *Acta Obstetrics et Gynecologica Scandinavica*, 87(7): 751–9.

Lindgren, H., Hildingsson, I. and Christensson, K. (2008b) Transfers in planned homebirths related to midwife availability and continuity: a nationwide population-based study. *Birth*, 25(1): 9–15.

LoCicero, A. (1993) Explaining excessive rates of cesareans and other childbirth interventions: contributions from contemporary theories of gender and psychosocial development. *Social Science & Medicine*, 37(10): 1261–9.

Long, L. (2003) Defining third stage of labour care and discussing optimal practice. *Midirs*, 13(3): 366–70.

Long, L. (2006) Redefining the second stage of labour could help to promote normal birth. *British Journal of Midwifery*, 14(2): 104–6.

Lothian, J. and DeVries, C. (2005) *The Official Lamaze Guide: Giving Birth with Confidence*. New York: Meadowbrook Press.

Low, L. and Moffat, A. (2006) Every labor is unique: but 'Call when your contractions are 3 minutes apart'. *MCN: The American Journal of Maternal/Child Health*, 31(5): 307–12.

Low, L., Seng, J., Murtland, T. and Oakley, D. (2000) Clinical: specific episiotomy rates – impact on perineal outcomes. *Journal of Midwifery & Women's Health*, 45(2): 87–93.

Lundquist, M., Olsson, A., Nissen, E. and Norman, M. (2000) Is it necessary to suture all lacerations after a vaginal delivery? *Birth*, 27(2): 79–85.

Luthy, D.A., Shy, K.K., van Belle, G., Larson, E.B., Hughes, J.P., Benedetti, T.J., Brown, Z.A., Effer, S., King, J.F. and Stenchever, M.A. (1987) A randomized trial of electronic fetal monitoring in preterm labor. *Obstetrics & Gynecology*, 69(5): 687–95.

Maassen, M., Hendrix, M., Van Vugt, H., Veersema, S., Smits, F. and Nijhuis, J.G. (2008) Operative deliveries in low-risk pregnancies in the Netherlands: primary versus secondary care. *Birth*, 35(4): 277–82.

MacArthur, C., Glazener, C., Lancashire, R. *et al.* (2005) Faecal incontinence and mode of first and subsequent delivery: a six year longitudinal study. *British Journal of Obstetrics and Gynaecology*, 112: 1075–82.

MacArthur, C., Glazener, C., Wilson, P., Herbison, G. *et al.* (2001) Obstetric practice and faecal incontinence three months after delivery. *British Journal of Obstetrics and Gynaecology*, 108: 678–83.

McCandlish, R., Bowler, U., van Asten, H., Berridge, G. *et al.* (1998) A randomised controlled trial of care of the perineum during second stage of normal labour. *British Journal of Obstetrics and Gynaecology*, 105: 1262–72.

McCourt, C. (ed.) (2010) *Childbirth, Midwifery and Concepts of Time*. London: Berghahn Books.

MacDonald, D. (1996) Cerebral palsy and intrapartum fetal monitoring. *New England Journal of Medicine*, 334(10): 659–60.

MacDonald, D., Grant, A. and Sheridan-Pereira, M. (1985) The Dublin randomized control trial of intrapartum fetal heart rate monitoring. *American Journal of Obstetrics & Gynecology*, 152(5): 524–39.

McDonald, G. (2010) Diagnosing the latent phase of labour: use of a partogram. *British Journal of Midwifery*, 18(10): 630–7.

McDonald, S. and Middleton, P. (2008) Effect of timing of umbilical cord clamping of term infants on maternal and neonatal outcomes. *Cochrane Database of Systematic Reviews*, Issue 2.

McDonald, S., Abbott, J.M. and Higgins, S.P. (2006) Prophylactic ergometrine-oxytocin versus oxytocin for the third stage of labour (Cochrane Review). In *The Cochrane Library*, Issue 3. Chichester: John Wiley & Sons, Ltd.

Machin, D. and Scamell, M. (1997) The experience of labour: using ethnography to explore the irresistible nature of the bio-medical metaphor during labour. *Midwifery*, 13: 78–84.

McInnes, R., Hillan, E., Clark, D. and Gilmour, H. (2004) Diamorphine for pain relief in labour: a randomised controlled trial comparing intramuscular injection and patient-controlled analgesia. *BJOG*, 1119(10): 1081–9.

Mack, S. (2000) Alexander Technique. In D. Tiran and S. Mack (eds) *Complementary Therapies for Pregnancy and Childbirth*. London: Bailliere Tindall.

McKay, S. (1991) Shared power: the essence of humanised childbirth. *Pre and Peri-Natal Psychology*, 5(4): 283–95.

MacKenzie, H. and van Teijlingen, E. (2010) Risk, theory, social and medical models: a critical analysis of the concept of risk in maternity care. *Midwifery*, 26: 488–96.

McLean, M., Thompson, D. and Zhang, H. (1994) Corticotrophin releasing hormone and beta-endorphin in labour. *European Journal of Endocrinology*, 131(2): 167–72.

MacLennan, A., Crowther, C. and Derham, R. (1994) Does the option to ambulate during spontaneous labour confer any advantage or disadvantage? *Journal of Maternal & Fetal Medicine*, 3(1): 43–8.

McMillan, A., Barlow, J. and Redshaw, M. (2009) *Birth and Beyond: A Review of the Evidence about Antenatal Education*. University of Warwick.

Madaan, M. and Trivedi, S. (2006) Intrapartum electronic fetal monitoring vs. intermittent auscultation in post caesarean pregnancies. *International Journal of Gynecology & Obstetrics*, 94: 123–5.

Maimburg, R., Væth, M., Dürr, J., Hvidman, L. and Olsen, J. (2010) Randomised trial of structured antenatal training sessions to improve the birth process. *BJOG*, 20(117): 921–8.

Mander, R. (2001) *Supportive Care and Midwifery*. Oxford: Blackwell Science.

Mander, R. (2002) The transitional stage. *The Practising Midwife*, 5(1): 10–12.

Mander, R. (2011) *Pain in Childbirth and Its Control*, 2nd edn. Oxford: Wiley-Blackwell.

Martensson, L. and Wallin, G. (2008) Sterile water injections as treatment for low-back pain during labour: a review. *Australian and New Zealand Journal of Obstetrics and Gynaecology*, 48: 369–74.

Martin, A., Schauble, P., Rai, S. and Curry, R. (2001) The effects of hypnosis on the labour processes and birth outcomes of pregnant adolescents. *Journal of Family Practice*, 50(5): 441–3.

Martin, E. (1987) *The Woman in the Body: A Cultural Analysis of Reproduction*. Milton Keynes: Open University Press.

Mason, L., Glenn, S., Walton, I. and Appleton, C. (1999a) The prevalence of stress incontinence during pregnancy and following birth. *Midwifery*, 15(2): 120–7.

Mason, L., Glenn, S., Walton, I. and Appleton, C. (1999b) The experience of stress incontinence after birth. *Birth*, 26(3): 164–71.

Matthews, A., Scott, P., Gallagher, P. and Corbally, M. (2006) An exploratory study of the conditions important in the facilitating the empowerment of midwives. *Midwifery*, 22(2): 181–91.

Maude, R. and Foureur, M. (2007) It's beyond water: stories of women's experience of using water for labour and birth. *Women & Birth*, 20: 17–24.

Mayerhofer, K., Bodner-Adler, B., Bodner, K. *et al.* (2002) Traditional care of the perineum during birth: a prospective randomised multi-centre study of 1,076 women. *Journal of Reproductive Medicine*, 47(6): 477–82.

Mead, M. (2008) Midwives' perspectives in 11 UK maternity units. In S. Downe (ed.) *Normal Childbirth: Evidence and Debate*. London: Churchill Livingstone.

Menage, J. (1996) Post-traumatic stress disorder following obstetric/gynaecological procedures. *British Journal of Midwifery*, 4(10): 532–3.

Menticoglou, S., Manning, F., Harman, C. *et al.* (1995) Perinatal outcome in relation to second stage duration. *American Journal of Obstetrics & Gynecology*, 173(3): 906–12.

Mercer, J. (2001) Current best evidence: a review of the literature on umbilical cord clamping. *Journal of Midwifery & Women's Health*, 46(6): 402–14.

Mercer, J. and Erikson-Owens, D. (2010) Evidence for neonatal transition and the first hour of life. In D. Walsh and S. Downe (eds) *Essential Midwifery Practice: Intrapartum Care*. London: Wiley-Blackwell.

Mercer, J. and Skovgaard, R. (2002) Neonatal transitional physiology: a new paradigm. *Journal of Perinatal and Neonatal Nursing*, 15(4): 56–75.

Metcalfe, A., Bick, D., Tohill, S., Williams, A. and Haldon, V. (2006) A prospective study of repair and non-repair of second-degree trauma: results and issues for future research. *Evidence Based Midwifery*, 4(2): 60–4.

Metcalfe, A., Tohill, S., Williams, A. *et al.* (2002) A pragmatic tool for the measurement of perineal tears. *British Journal of Midwifery*, 10: 412–17.

Meyer, S., Weible, C. and Woeber, K. (2010) Perceptions and practice of waterbirth: a survey of Georgia midwives. *Journal of Midwifery & Women's Health*, 55: 55–9.

Michel, S., Rake, A., Treiber, K. *et al.* (2002) MR obstetric pelvimetry: effects of birthing position on pelvic bony dimensions. *American Journal of Roentgenology*, 179: 1063–7.

Middle, J. and Wee, Y. (2009) Informed consent for epidural analgesia in labour: a survey of UK practice. *Anaesthesia*, 64: 161–4.

*Midirs* and the NHS Centre for Reviews and Dissemination (2004) *Positions in Labour and Delivery*. Informed Choice for Professionals Leaflet.

Milan, M. (2003) Childbirth as healing: three women's experience of independent midwife care. *Complementary Therapies in Nursing & Midwifery*, 9: 140–6.

Milewa, T. and Barry, C. (2005) Health policy and the politics of evidence. *Social Policy and Administration*, 39(5): 498–512.

Miller, J. and Petrie, J. (2000) Development of practice guidelines. *Lancet*, 355(9198): 82–3.

Mitchell, M. and Williams, J. (2006) Integrating complementary therapies. *The Practising Midwife*, 9(3): 12–15.

Moberg, K. (2004) *The Oxytocin Factor*. New York: Perseus Books.

Money, M. (1997) Shamanism and complementary therapy. *Complementary Therapies in Nursing & Midwifery*, 6: 207–12.

Mongan, M. (2005) *HypnoBirthing: The Mongan Method*. Deerfield Beach, FL: Health Communication, Inc.

Moore, E.R., Anderson, G.C. and Bergman, N. (2007) Early skin-to-skin contact for mothers and their healthy newborn infants. *Cochrane Database of Systematic Reviews*, Issue 3.

Moorhead, J. (2004, 8 Spetember) The home birth lottery. *Guardian*. Online: www.guardian. co.uk/lifeandstyle/2004/sep/08/familyandrelationships.health.

Morkved, S., Bo K., Schei, B. and Salvesen, K. (2003) Pelvic floor muscle training during pregnancy to prevent urinary incontinence: a single-blind randomised controlled trial. *Obstetrics & Gynecology*, 101: 313–19.

Mota, R., Costa, F., Amaral, A. *et al.* (2009) Skin adhesive versus subcuticular for perineal skin repair after episiotomy: a randomised controlled trial. *Acta Obstetrics Gynaecologica*, 88: 660–6.

Motha, G. and McGrath, J. (1993) The effects of reflexology on labour outcomes. *Journal of the Association of Reflexologists*, 2–4.

Mottershead, N. (2006) Hypnosis: removing the labour from birth. *The Practising Midwife*, 9(3): 26–9.

Mousely, S. (2005) Audit of an aromatherapy service in a maternity unit. *Complementary Therapies in Clinical Practice*, 11: 205–10.

Munro, J., Ford, H. and Scott, A. (2002) Action research project responding to midwives views of different methods of fetal monitoring in labour. *Midirs*, 12(4): 492–5.

Munro, J., Soltani, H., Layhe, N., Watts, K. and Hughes A. (2004) Can women relate to the midwifery behind the machines? An exploration of women's experience of electronic fetal monitoring: cross-sectional survey in three hospitals. Normal Labour and Birth: 2nd Research Conference, 9–11 June; University of Central Lancashire.

Murphy-Lawless, J. (1998) *Reading Birth and Death: A History of Obstetric Thinking*. Cork: Cork University Press.

Myles, T. and Santolaya, J. (2003) Maternal and neonatal outcomes in patients with a prolonged second stage of labour. *Obstetrics & Gynecology*, 102: 52–8.

Myrfield, K., Brook, C. and Creedy, D. (1997) Reducing perineal trauma: implications of flexion and extension of the fetal head during birth. *Midwifery* 13(4): 197–201.

NCT (2010) www.nct.org.uk/home.

Neal, J., Lowe, N., Patrick, T., Cabbage, L. and Corwin, E. (2010) What is the slowest-yet-normal cervical dilation rate among nulliparous women with spontaneous labour onset? *Journal of Obstetric, Gynecologic, & Neonatal Nursing*, 39: 361–9.

Neilson, J.P. (2006) Fetal electrocardiogram (ECG) for fetal monitoring during labour. *Cochrane Database of Systematic Reviews*, Issue 3.

Neisheim, B., Kinge, R., Berg, R. *et al.* (2003) Acupuncture during labour can reduce the use of Merperidine: a controlled study. *The Clinical Journal of Pain*, 19(3): 187–91.

Nelson, K., Dambrosia, J., Ting, T. and Grether, J. (1996) Uncertain value of electronic fetal monitoring in predicting cerebral palsy. *New England Journal of Medicine*, 334: 659–60.

Nettleton, S., Burrows, R. and Watt, I. (2008) Regulating medical bodies? The consequences of the 'modernisation' of the NHS and the disembodiment of clinical knowledge. *Sociology of Health & Illness*, 30(3): 333–48.

Neumark, J., Hammerle, A. and Biegelmayer, C. (1985) Effects of epidural anaesthesia on plasma catecholamines and cortisol in parturition. *Acta Anaesthesia Scandinavia*, 29(6): 555–9.

Newburn, M. and Singh, D. (2004) *Creating a Better Birth Environment: An Audit Toolkit*. London: NCT.

NICE (2007) *Guideline for Intrapartum Care*. Online: www.nice.org.uk (accessed 3 August 2006).

Niven, C. and Murphy-Black, T. (2000) Memory for labour pain: a review of the literature. *Birth*, 27(4): 254–5.

Nolan, M. (2005) Childbirth and parenting education: what the research says and why we may ignore it. In M. Nolan and J. Foster (eds) *Birth and Parenting Skills: New Directions in Antenatal Education*. London: Churchill Livingstone.

Nordstrom, L., Achanna, S., Naka, K. and Arulkumaran, S. (2001) Fetal and maternal lactate increase during active second stage of labour. *British Journal of Obstetrics and Gynaecology*, 108: 263–8.

Noren, H., Blad, S., Carlsson, A. *et al.* (2006) STAN in clinical practice: the outcome of 2 years of regular use in the city of Gothenburg. *American Journal of Obstetrics & Gynecology*, 195: 7–15.

North Staffordshire Changing Childbirth Research Team (2000) A randomised study of midwifery caseload care and traditional 'shared-care'. *Midwifery*, 16(4): 295–302.

NPEU (2011) *Birthplace*. Online: www.npeu.ox.ac.uk/birthplace (accessed 20 June 2011).

NPEU (2011) *INFANT*. Online: www.npeu.ox.ac.uk/infant (accessed November 2010).

Oakley, A. (1981) Interviewing women: a contradiction in terms. In H. Roberts (ed.) *Doing Feminist Research*. London: Routledge.

Oboro, V., Tabowei, T., Logo, O. and Bosah, J. (2003) A multi-centre evaluation of the two-layered repair of postpartum perineal trauma. *Journal of Obstetrics & Gynaecology*, 23(1): 5–8.

O'Brien, M.A., Freemantle, N., Oxman, A.D., Wolf, F., Davis, D.A. and Herrin, J. (2006) Continuing education meetings and workshops: effects on professional practice and health care outcomes (Cochrane Review). In *The Cochrane Library*, Issue 3. Chichester: John Wiley & Sons, Ltd.

O'Brien, M.A., Rogers, S., Jamtvedt, G., Oxman, A.D., Odgaard-Jensen, J., Kristoffersen, D.T., Forsetlund, L., Bainbridge, D., Freemantle, N., Davis, D., Haynes, R.B. and Harvey, E. (2007) Educational outreach visits: effects on professional practice and health care outcomes. *Cochrane Database of Systematic Reviews*, Issue 4.

Observer (2009, 12 July) It's good for women to suffer the pain of a natural birth, says medical chief. Online: www.guardian.co.uk/lifeandstyle/2009/jul/12/pregnancy-pain-natural-birth-yoga.

Odent, M. (2001) New reasons and new ways to study birth physiology. *International Journal of Gynecology & Obstetrics*, 75: S39–S45.

Odent, M. (2002) The first hour following birth: don't wake the mother. *Midwifery Today*, 61: 9–12.

O'Driscoll, K. and Meagher, D. (1986) *Active Management of Labour*. London: W.B. Saunders.

Olsen, O. (1997) Meta-analysis of the safety of home birth. *Birth*, 24(1): 4–13.

Olsen, O. and Jewell, M.D. (2009) Home versus hospital birth. *Cochrane Database of Systematic Reviews*, Issue 2.

Oscarsson, M., Amer-Wahlin, I., Rydhstroem, H. and Kallen, K. (2006) Outcome in obstetric care related to oxytocin use: a population-based study. *Acta Obstetrics et Gynaecologica*, 85(9): 1094–8.

Page, L., McCourt, C., Beake, S. and Hewison, J. (1999) Clinical interventions and outcomes of one-to-one midwifery practice. *Journal of Public Health Medicine*, 21(3): 243–8.

Pantoja, T., Romero, A., Green, M.E., Wyatt, J., Grimshaw, J., Denig, P., Durieux, P., Gill, P., Gordon, R., Haaijer Ruskamp, F., Hicks, N., Rowe, R. and Colomer, N. (2004) Manual paper reminders: effects on professional practice and health care outcomes. *Cochrane Database of Systematic Reviews*, Issue 2.

Parnell, C., Langhoff-Roos, J., Iverson, R. *et al.* (1993) Pushing method in the expulsive phase of labour: a randomised trial. *Acta Obstetrica et Gynecologica Scandinavia*, 72(1): 31–5.

Parr, M. (1997). *Description of a Study Evaluating a New Approach to Preparation for Parenting for Women and Men in the Transition to Parenthood* (Hertfordshire Longitudinal Study, 1989–93). Unpublished report.

Parratt, J. and Fahy, K. (2008) Including the nonrational in sensible midwifery. *Women and Birth*, 21: 37–42.

Paulson, J. and Bazemore, S. (2010) Prenatal and postpartum depression in fathers and its association with maternal depression: a meta-analysis. *Journal of American Medical Association*, 303(19): 1961–9.

Peleg, D., Kennedy, C.M., Merrill, D. and Zlatnik, M. (1999) Risk of repetition of a severe perineal laceration. *Obstetrics & Gynecology*, 93(6): 1021–4.

Pembroke, N.F. and Pembroke, J.J. (2008) The spirituality of presence in midwifery care. *Midwifery*, 24: 321–7.

Perkins, B. (2004) *The Medical Delivery Business: Health Reform, Childbirth and the Economic Order*. London: Rutgers University Press.

Philpott, R. and Castle, W. (1972) Cervicographs in the management of labour on primigravidae 1: the alert line for detecting abnormal labour. *Journal of Obstetrics & Gynaecology of the British Commonwealth*, 79: 592–8.

Piquard, F., Schaefer, A., Hsuing, R. *et al.* (1989) Are there two biological parts in the second stage of labour? *Acta Obstetrics et Gynaecologica*, 68(8): 713–18.

Polanyi, M. (1994) *Personal Knowledge: Towards a Post-critical Philosophy*. London: Routledge & Kegan Paul.

Ponkey, S., Cohen, A., Heffner, L. and Lieberman, E. (2003) Persistent fetal occiput posterior position: obstetric outcomes. *Obstetrics & Gynecology*, 101(5): 915–20.

Pope, C. (2003) Resisting evidence: the study of evidence-based medicine as a contemporary social movement. *Health. An Interdisciplinary Journal for the Social Study of Health, Illness & Medicine*, 7(3): 267–82.

Porter, S., Crozier, K., Sinclair, M. and Kernohan, W. (2007) New midwifery? A qualitative analysis of midwives' decision-making strategies. *Journal of Advanced Nursing*, 60(5): 525–34.

Posnett, J. (1999) Is bigger better? Concentration in the provision of secondary care. *British Medical Journal*, 319: 1063–5.

Rabe, H., Reynolds, G. and Diaz-Rossello, J. (2006) Early versus delayed umbilical cord clamping in preterm infants. *The Cochrane Database of Systematic Reviews*, Issue 3.

Ragnar, I., Altman, D., Tyden, T. and Olsson, S.E. (2006) Comparison of the maternal experience and duration of labour in two upright delivery positions: a randomised controlled trial. *BJOG*, 113: 165–70.

Rahm, V., Hallgren, A. and Hogberg, H. (2002) Plasma oxytocin levels in women during labor with or without epidural analgesia: a prospective study. *Acta Obstetricia et Gynecologica Scandinavica*, 81: 1033–9.

Rahnama, P., Ziaei, S. and Faghihzadeh, S. (2006) Impact of early admission in labour on method of delivery. *International Journal of Gynecology & Obstetrics*, 92: 217–20.

Raisanen, S., Vehvilainen-Julkunen, K. and Heinonen, S. (2009) The increased incidence of obstetric anal sphincter rupture: an emerging trend in Finland. *Preventive Medicine*, 49: 535–40.

Raisanen, S., Vehvilainen-Julkunen, K. and Heinonen, S. (2010) Need for can consequences for episiotomy in vaginal birth: a critical approach. *Midwifery*, 26: 348–56.

Rajan, L. (1994) The impact of obstetric procedures and analgesia/anaesthesia during labour and delivery on breastfeeding. *Midwifery*, 10(2): 87–102.

Ramesh, R. (2010, 16 August) Midwives attack hysteria over home births. *Guardian*. www.guardian.co.uk/lifeandstyle/2010/aug/16/homebirths-midwives-hospital-baby.

Ramnero, A., Hanson, U. and Kihlgren, M. (2002) Acupuncture treatment during labour: a randomised controlled trial. *British Journal of Obstetrics and Gynaecology*, 109: 637–44.

Ransjo-Arvidson, A., Matthiesen, A., Lilja, G. *et al.* (2001) Maternal analgesia during labour disturbs newborn behaviour: effects on breastfeeding, temperature and crying. *Birth*, 23(3): 136–43.

Razgaitis, E.J. and Lyvers, A.N. (2010) Management of protracted active labor with nipple stimulation: a viable tool for midwives? *Journal of Midwifery & Women's Health*, 55: 65–9.

Read, J., Miller, F. and Paul, R. (1981) Randomized trial of ambulation versus oxytocin for labor enhancement: a preliminary report. *American Journal of Obstetrics & Gynecology*, 139: 669–72.

Reddy, K., Reginald, P., Spring, J., Nunn, L. and Mishra, N. (2004) A free-standing low-risk maternity unit in the United Kingdom: does it have a role? *Journal of Obstetrics & Gynaecology*, 24(4): 360–6.

Redshaw, M., Rowe, R., Hockley, C. and Brocklehurst, P. (2006) *Recorded Delivery: A National Survey of Women's Experience of Maternity Care*. Oxford: NPEU.

Regan, M. and Liaschenko, J. (2007) In the mind of the beholder: hypothesized effect of intrapartum nurses' cognitive frames of childbirth caesarean section rate. *Qualitative Health Research*, 17(5): 612–24.

Reichman, O., Gdansky, E. and Latinsky, B. (2007) Digital rotation from occipto-posterior to occipto-anterior decreases need for caesarean section. *European Journal of Obstetrics & Gynecology and Reproductive Biology*, 136: 25–8.

Report of the Maternity Services Review (2009) *Improving Maternity Services in Australia*. Canberra: Federal Government.

Ribeiro, S., Kennedy, S. and Smith, R. (2005) Interface of physical and emotional stress regulation through endogenous opioid system and mu-opioid receptors. *Progress in Neuropsychopharmacological Biological Psychiatry*, 29(8): 1264–80.

Richens, Y. (2002) Are midwives using research evidence in practice? *British Journal of Midwifery*, 10(1): 11–16.

Richter, H., Brumfield, C., Cliver, S., Burgio, K. *et al.* (2002) Risk factors associated with anal sphincter tear: a comparison of primiparous patients, vaginal births after caesarean deliveries and patients with previous vaginal delivery. *American Journal of Obstetrics & Gynecology*, 187: 1194–8.

Ridley, R. (2007) Diagnosis and intervention for occiput posterior malposition. *Journal of Obstetric, Gynecologic, & Neonatal Nursing*, 36: 135–43.

Rizk, D. and Thomas, L. (2000) Relationship between the length of the perineum and position of the anus and vaginal delivery in primigravidae. *International Urogynecology Journal*, 11: 79–83.

Roberts, J. (2002) The 'push' for evidence: management of the second stage. *Journal of Midwifery & Women's Health*, 47(1): 2–15.

Roberts, J. (2003) A new understanding of the second stage of labour: implications for nursing care. *Journal of Obstetric, Gynecologic, & Neonatal Nursing*, 32(6): 794–801.

Roberts, L., Gulliver, B., Fisher, J. and Cloyes, K. (2010) The coping with labor algorithm: an alternate pain assessment tool for the labouring woman. *Journal of Midwifery & Women's Health*, 55: 107–16.

Robertson, A. (1997) *The Midwife Companion*. Sydney: Ace Graphics.

Robohm, J. and Buttenheim, M. (1996) The gynaecological care experience of adult survivors of childhood sexual abuse: a preliminary investigation. *Women & Health*, 24(3): 59–75.

Rogers, E. (1995) *The Diffusion of Innovations*, 4th edn. New York: Free Press.

Rogers, R., Leeman, L., Migliaccio, L. and Albers, L. (2008) Does the severity of spontaneous genital tract trauma affect postpartum pelvic floor function? *International Urogynecology Journal*, 19: 429–35.

Rogers, W. (2004) Evidence-based medicine and women: do the principles and practice of EBM further women's health? *Bioethics*, 18(1): 50–72.

Rogerson, L., Mason, G. and Roberts, A. (2000) Preliminary experience with twenty perineal repairs using Indermil tissue adhesive. *European Journal of Obstetrics & Gynecology and Reproductive Biology*, 88: 139–42.

Romero, A., Green, M., Pantoja, T., Watt, J. *et al.* (2006) Manuel paper reminders: effects on professional practice and health care outcomes (Cochrane Review). In *The Cochrane Library*, Issue 3. Chichester: John Wiley & Sons, Ltd.

Rortveit, G., Daltveit, A., Hannestad, Y. and Hunskaar, S. (2003) Vaginal delivery parameters and urinary incontinence: the Norwegian EPINCONT study. *American Journal of Obstetrics & Gynecology*, 189: 1268–74.

Rortveit, G., Kjersti, D., Yugvild, S., Hannestad, S. and Hunskaar S. (2003) Urinary incontinence after vaginal delivery or caesarean section. *New England Journal of Medicine*, 348: 900–7.

Rosen, M. (2002) Nitrous oxide for relief of labour pain: a systematic review. *American Journal of Obstetrics & Gynecology*, 186: S110–26.

Rosen, P. (2004) Supporting women in labour: analysis of different types of caregivers. *Journal of Midwifery & Women's Health*, 49(1): 24–31.

Rosenberg, K. and Trevathan, W. (2003) Birth, obstetrics and human evolution. *British Journal of Obstetrics and Gynaecology*, 109(11): 1199–206.

Rossiter-Thornton, J. (2002) Prayer in your practice. *Complementary Therapies in Nursing & Midwifery*, 8: 21–8.

Rouse, D., Weiner, S., Bloom, S., Varner, M. and Spong, C. (2009) Second stage labor duration in nulliparous women: relationship to maternal and perinatal outcomes. *American Journal of Obstetrics & Gynecology*, 201: 357.e1–7.

Rowe, R. (2010) Local guidelines for the transfer of women from midwifery unit to obstetric unit during labour in England: a systematic appraisal of their quality. *Quality and Safety in Health Care*, 19: 90–4.

Royal College of Midwives (2006) *Campaign for Normal Birth*. Online: www.rcmnormalbirth.org.uk/default.asp?sID=1099658666156 (accessed 6 August 2006).

Royal College of Nursing (1998) *Evidence-based Care in Nursing*. London: RCN.

Royal College of Obstetricians and Gynaecologist (RCOG) (2007) *Management of Third and Fourth Degree Perineal Tears Used in Perineal Care*. Guideline no. 29. London: RCOG.

Ruckhaberle, E., Jundt, K., Bauerle, M. *et al.* (2009) Prospective randomised controlled trial with the birth trainer EPI-NO for the prevention of perineal trauma. *Australian and New Zealand Journal of Obstetrics and Gynaecology*, 49: 478–83.

Russell, K. (forthcoming) Struggling to get into the pool room? A critical discourse analysis of labour ward midwives experiences of water birth. Accepted for publication in *International Journal of Childbirth*.

Ryding, E., Wijma, K. and Wijma, B. (1998) Experiences of emergency caesarean section: a phenomenological study of 53 women. *Birth*, 25(4): 246–51.

Sackett, D. (1996) Evidence based medicine: what it is and what it isn't. *British Medical Journal*, 312: 71–2.

Salamalekis, E., Siristatidis, C., Vasios, G., Saloum, J. *et al.* (2006) Fetal pulse oximetry and wavelet analysis of the fetal heart rate in the evaluation of abnormal cardiotocography tracings. *Journal of Obstetric and Gynaecology Research*, 32(2): 135–9.

Salmon, D. (1999) A feminist analysis of women's experiences of perineal trauma in the immediate post-delivery period. *Midwifery*, 15(4): 247–56.

Sampselle, C. (2000) Behavioural intervention for urinary incontinence in women: evidence for practice. *Journal of Midwifery & Women's Health* 45(2): 94–103.

Sampselle, C. and Hines, S. (1999) Spontaneous pushing during birth: relationship to perineal outcomes. *Journal of Midwifery & Women's Health*, 44(1): 36–9.

Sampselle, C., Miller, J., Luecha, Y., Fischer, K. and Rosten, L. (2005) Provider support of spontaneous pushing during the second stage of labour. *Journal of Obstetric, Gynecologic, & Neonatal Nursing*, 34: 695–702.

Sandall, J. (1997) Midwives' burnout and continuity of care. *British Journal of Midwifery*, 5(2): 106–11.

Sanders, J., Campbell, R. and Peters, T. (2002) Effectiveness of pain relief during perineal suturing. *British Journal of Obstetrics and Gynaecology*, 109: 1066–8.

Sanson-Fisher, R. (2004) Diffusion of innovation theory for clinical change. *Medical Journal of Australia*, 180: S55–S56.

Sartore, A., De Seta, F., Maso, G. *et al.* (2004) The effects of mediolateral episiotomy on pelvic floor function after vaginal delivery. *Obstetrics & Gynecology*, 103: 669–73.

Sartore, A., Pregazzi, R. and Bortolli, P. (2003) Effects of epidural analgesia during labor on pelvic floor function after vaginal delivery. *Acta Obstetricia et Gynecologica Scandinavica*, 82: 143–6.

Saunders, N., Paterson, C. and Wadsworth, J. (1992) Neonatal and maternal morbidity in relation to the length of the second stage of labour. *British Journal of Obstetrics and Gynaecology*, 99(5): 381–5.

Scarabotto, L. and Riesco, M. (2008) Use of hyaluronidase to prevent perineal trauma during spontaneous delivery: a pilot study. *Journal of Midwifery & Women's Health*, 53: 353–61.

Schaffer, J., Bloom, S., Casey, B. *et al.* (2005) A randomized trial of the effect of coached vs uncoached maternal pushing during the second stage of labor on postpartum pelvic floor structure and function. *American Journal of Obstetrics & Gynecology*, 192: 1692–6.

Scheller, J. and Nelson, K. (1994) Does caesarean delivery prevent cerebral palsy or other neurological problems of childhood? *Obstetrics & Gynecology*, 83(4): 624–30.

Schiermeier, S., Pildner von Steinburg, S., Thieme, A., Reinhard, J., Daumer, M., Scholz, M., Hatzmann, W. and Schneider K. (2008) Sensitivity and specificity of intrapartum computerised FIGO criteria for cardiotocography and fetal scalp pH during labour: multicentre, observational study. *BJOG*, 115: 1557–63.

Schon, D. (1995) Knowing-in-action: the new scholarship requires a new epistemology. *Change*, 27(6): 26–34.

Scott, T., Mannion, R., Marshall, M. and Davies, H. (2003) Does organisational culture influence health care performance? A review of the evidence. *Journal of Health Service Research & Policy*, 8(2): 105–17.

Scupholme, A. and Kamons, A. (1987) Are outcomes compromised when mothers are assigned to birth centres for care? *Journal of Nurse Midwifery*, 4: 211–15.

Shallow, H. (2003) My rolling programme: the birth ball – ten years experience of using the physiotherapy ball for labouring women. *Midirs*, 13: 28–30.

Shaw, B., Cheater, F., Baker, R., Gillies, C., Hearnshaw, H., Flottorp, S. and Robertson, N. (2006) Tailored interventions to overcome identified barriers to change: effects on professional practice and health care outcomes. *The Cochrane Database of Systematic Reviews*, Issue 3.

Shepherd, A., Cheyne, H. and Kennedy, S. (2010) The purple line as a measure of labour progress: a longitudinal study. *BMC Pregnancy and Childbirth*, 10:54.

Shipman, M., Boniface, D., Tefft, M. and McCloghry, F. (1997) Antenatal perineal massage and subsequent perineal outcomes: a randomised controlled trial. *British Journal of Obstetrics and Gynaecology*, 104: 787–91.

Shorten, A., Donsante, J. and Shorten, B. (2002) Birth position, accoucheur and perineal outcomes: informing women about choices for vaginal birth. *Birth*, 29(1): 1827.

Shribman, S. (2007) *Making It Better: For Mother and Baby – Clinical Case for Change*. London: Department of Health.

Sidenbladh, E. (1983) *Water Babies: A Book about Igor Tjarkovsky and His Method for Delivering and Training Children in Water*. London: St Martins.

Simkin, P. (1989) Non-pharmacological methods of pain relief during labour. In I. Chalmers, M. Enkin and M. Kierse (eds) *Effective Care in Pregnancy and Childbirth*. Oxford: Oxford University Press.

Simkin, P. (2010) The fetal occiput posterior position: state of science and a new perspective. *Birth*, 37(1): 61–71.

Simkin, P. and Ancheta, R. (2005) *The Labour Progress Handbook*, 2nd edn. London: Blackwell Science.

Simkin, P. and Ancheta, R. (2011) *The Labour Progress Handbook*, 3rd edn. Oxford: Blackwell Science.

Simkin, P. and O'Hara, M. (2002) Non-pharmacological relief of pain during labor: systematic review of five methods. *American Journal of Obstetrics & Gynecology*, 186: S131–59.

Simmons, S., Dennis, A., Cyna, A. and Hughes D. (2008) Combined spinal-epidural versus epidural analgesia in labour (Cochrane Review). In *The Cochrane Library*, Issue 1. Chichester: John Wiley & Sons.

Simpson, K. and James, D. (2005) Effects of immediate versus delayed pushing during second-stage labour on fetal well-being. *Nursing Research*, 54(3): 149–57.

Skilnand, E., Fossen, D. and Heiberg, E. (2002) Acupuncture in the management of pain in labour. *Acta Obstetrica et Gynaecologica Scandinavica*, 81(10): 943–8.

Sleep, J., Grant, A., Garcia, J., Elbourne, D., Spencer, J. and Chalmers, I. (1984) West Berkshire perineal management trial. *British Medical Journal*, 289: 587–90.

Smith, C.A., Collins, C.T., Cyna, A.M. and Crowther, C.A. (2006) Complementary and alternative therapies for pain management in labour. *Cochrane Database of Systematic Reviews*, Issue 4.

Smith, L. and Smith C. (2005). UK childbirth delivery options in 2001–2002: alternatives to consultant unit booking and delivery. *British Journal of General Practice*, 55: 292–7.

Smith, M., Acheson, L., Byrd, J. *et al.* (1991) A critical review of labour and birth care. *Journal of Family Practice*, 35: 107–15.

Smyth, R.M.D., Alldred, S.K. and Markham, C. (2008) Amniotomy for shortening spontaneous labour. *Cochrane Database of Systematic Reviews*, Issue 4.

Soltani, H., Dickinson, F. and Symonds, I. (2006) Placental cord drainage after spontaneous vaginal delivery as part of the management of the third stage of labour. *Cochrane Database of Systematic Reviews*, Issue 3.

Soltani, H., Hutchon, D. and Poulose, T. (2010) Timing of prophylactic uterotonics for the third stage of labour after vaginal birth. *Cochrane Database of Systematic Reviews*, Issue 8.

Sookhoo, M. and Biott, C. (2002) Learning at work: midwives judging progress in labour. *Learning in Health & Social Care*, 1(2): 75–85.

Soong, B. and Barnes, M. (2005) Maternal position at midwife-attended birth and perineal trauma: is there an association? *Birth*, 3: 164–9.

Speca, M., Carlson, L., Goodey, E. and Angen, M. (2000) A randomised, wait-list controlled clinical trial: the effects of a mindfulness meditation-based stress reduction program on mood and symptoms of stress in cancer patients. *Psychosomatic Medicine*, 62: 613–22.

Spencer, S. (2005) Giving birth on the beach: hypnosis and psychology. *The Practising Midwife*, 8(1): 27–9.

Spiby, H. and Munro, J. (2010) *Evidence Based Midwifery: Applications in Context*. London: Wiley-Blackwell.

Spiby, H., Slade, P., Escott, D., Henderson, B. and Fraser, R. (2003) Selected coping strategies in labour: an investigation of women's experiences. *Birth*, 30: 189–94.

Spintge, R. (1989) Some neuro-endocrinological effects of so-called anxiolytic music. *International Journal of Neurology*, 19/20, 186–96.

Spitzer, M. (1995) Birth centres: economy, safety and empowerment. *Journal of Nurse-Midwifery*, 40(4) (July/August): 371–5.

Stafford, S. (2001) Is lack of autonomy a reason for leaving midwifery? *The Practising Midwife*, 4(7): 46–7.

Stamp, G., Kruzins, G. and Crowther, C. (2001) Perineal massage in labour and prevention of perineal trauma: randomised controlled trial. *British Medical Journal*, 322: 1277–80.

Stapleton, H. and Tiran, D. (2000) Herbal medicine. In D. Tiran and S. Mack (eds) *Complementary Therapies for Pregnancy and Childbirth*. London: Bailliere Tindall.

Stapleton, H., Kirkham, M., Thomas, G. and Curtis, P. (2002) Midwives in the middle: balance and vulnerability. *British Journal of Midwifery*, 10(10): 607–11.

Stark, M. and Miller, M. (2009) Barriers to the use of hydrotherapy in labor. *Journal of Obstetric, Gynecologic, & Neonatal Nursing*, 38: 667–75.

Stark, M., Rudell, B. and Haus, G. (2008) Observing position and movement in hydrotherapy: a pilot study. *Journal of Obstetric, Gynecologic, & Neonatal Nursing*, 37: 116–22.

Steen, M., Cooper, K., Marchant, P. *et al.* (2000) A randomised controlled trial to compare the effectiveness of icepacks and Epifoam with cooling maternity gel pads at alleviating postnatal perineal trauma. *Midwifery*, 16: 48–55.

Stewart, J., Andrews, J. and Cartlidge, P. (1998) Number of deaths related to intrapartum asphyxia and timing of death in Wales perinatal survey. *British Medical Journal*, 316: 657–60.

Stewart, M. (2001) Whose evidence counts? An exploration of health professional perceptions of evidence-based practice focusing on maternity services. *Midwifery*, 17(4): 279–88.

Stewart, M. (2005) 'I'm just going to wash you down': sanitizing the vaginal examination. *Journal of Advanced Nursing*, 51(6): 587–94.

Stewart, M., McCandlish, R. and Henderson, J. (2004) *Report of a Structured Review of Birth Centre Outcomes*. Oxford: NPEU.

Stocks, L., Rowland, J. and Martindale, E. (2010) The use of the birthing pool after diagnosis of stillbirth. *Journal of Obstetrics & Gynaecology*, 30(2): 200.

Stockton, A. (2003) Homeopathy as an integral part of maternity care – why not? *RCM Midwives News & Appointments*, April, 6–7.

Stremler, R., Hodnett, E., Petryshen, P. *et al.* (2005) Randomized controlled trial of hands-and-knees positioning for occipitoposterior position in labour. *Birth*, 32(4): 243–51.

Stuart, C. (2000) Invasive actions in labour: where have all the old tricks gone? *The Practising Midwife*, 3(8): 30–3.

Studd, J. (1973) Partograms and nomograms of cervical dilatation in management of primi-gravid labour. *British Medical Journal*, 4: 451–5.

Sutton, J. (2001) *Let Birth Be Born Again*. Middlesex: Birth Concepts UK.

Sutton, J. and Scott, P. (1996) *Understanding and Teaching Optimal Fetal Positioning*. Tauranga, New Zealand: Birth Concepts.

Symon, A., Winter, C., Inkster, M. and Donnan, P. (2009) Outcomes for births booked under maternity units: matched comparison study independent midwife and births in NHS. *British Medical Journal*, 338: 2060.

Taylor, S. (1990) Oxytocin. In R. Palmeira (ed.) *In the Gold of Flesh: Poems of Birth and Motherhood*. London: The Women's Press.

Taylor, S., Klein, L., Lewis, B., Gruenewald, T., Gurung, R. and Updegraff, J. (2000) Biobeha-vioural responses to stress in females: tend-and-befriend, not fight-or-flight. *Psychological Review*, 107(3): 411–29.

Teate, A., Leap, N., Schindler Rising, S. and Homer, C. (2009) Women's experiences of group antenatal care in Australia: the CenteringPregnancy pilot study. *Midwifery*: doi:10.1016/j. midw.2009.03.001.

Terry, R., Westcott, J., O'Shea, L. and Kelly, F. (2006) Postpartum outcomes in supine position by physicians vs nonsupine delivery by midwives. *JAOA*, 106(4): 199–202.

Tew, M. (1998) *Safer Childbirth? A Critical History of Maternity Care*. London: Chapman & Hall.

Thacker, S.B., Stroup, D. and Chang, M.H. (2006) Continuous electronic heart rate monitoring for fetal assessment during labor. *Cochrane Database of Systematic Reviews*, Issue 3.

Thomas, T. (2001) Becoming a mother: matrescence as spiritual formation. *Religious Education*, 96(1): 88–105.

Thomson, A. (1993) Pushing techniques in the second stage of labour. *Journal of Advanced Nursing*, 18: 171–7.

Thomson, G. and Downe, S. (2010) Changing the future to change the past: women's experience of a psotivie birth experience following a traumatic birth experience. *Journal of Reproductive and Infant Psychology*, 28(1): 102–12.

Thöni, A., Zech, N. and Ploner F. (2007) Giving birth in the water: experience after 1,825 water deliveries – retrospective descriptive comparison of water birth and traditional delivery methods. *Gynakol Geburtshilfliche Rundsch*, 47(2): 76–80.

Thorgen, A. and Crang-Svalenius, E. (2009) Birth centre in the East Midlands: views and experiences of midwives. *British Journal of Midwifery*, 17(3): 144–51.

Tiran, D. and Mack, S. (2000) *Complementary Therapies for Pregnancy and Childbirth*. London: Bailliere Tindall.

Torvaldsen, S., Roberts, C. and Bell, J., Raynes-Greenow, C. (2006) Discontinuation of epidural analgesia late in labour for reducing the adverse delivery outcomes associated with epidural analgesia. *Cochrane Database of Systematic Reviews*, Issue 2.

Tracey, S., Sullivan, E. and Wang, Y. (2007) Birth outcomes associated with intervention in labour amongst low risk women: a population-based study. *Women & Birth*, 20(2): 41–8.

Tracy, S. and Tracy, M. (2003) Costing the cascade: estimating the cost of increased obstetric intervention in childbirth using population data. *BJOG*, 110(8): 717–24.

Trutnovsky, G., Haas, J., Lang, U. and Petru, E. (2006) Women's perception of sexuality during pregnancy and after birth. *Australian and New Zealand Journal of Obstetrics and Gynaecology*, 46: 282–7.

Turnbull, D., Holmes, S., Cheyne, H. *et al.* (1996) Randomised controlled trial of efficacy of midwifery-managed care. *Lancet*, 348: 213–18.

Ullman, R., Smith, L., Burns, E., Mori, R. and Dowswell, T. (2010) Parenteral opioids for maternal pain relief in labour. *Cochrane Database of Systematic Reviews*, Issue 9.

Uvnas-Moberg, K. (2003). *The Oxytocin Factor: Tapping the Hormone of Calm, Love and Healing*. Cambridge, MA: Da Capo Press.

van Ham M., van Dongen, P. and Mulder, J. (1997) Maternal consequences of caesarean section: a retrospective study of intra-operative and postoperative maternal complications of caesarean section during a 10 year period. *European Journal of Obstetrics & Gynecology and Reproductive Biology*, 74(1): 1–6.

Van Teijlingen, E. (2005) A critical analysis of the medical model as used in the study of pregnancy and childbirth. *Sociological Research Online*, 10(2): www.socresonline.org.uk/10/2/teijlingen.html (accessed February 2008).

Veeramah, V. (2004) Utilisation of research findings by graduate nurses and midwives. *Journal of Advanced Nursing*, 47(2): 183–91.

Viisainen, K. (2001) Negotiating control and meaning: home birth as a self-constructed choice in Finland. *Social Science & Medicine*, 52(7): 1109–21.

Wagner, M. (2001) Fish can't see water: the need to humanize birth. *International Journal of Gynecology & Obstetrics*, 75: S25–S37.

Walker, D. and Worrell, R. (2008) Promoting healthy pregnancies through perinatal groups: a comparison of CenterPregnancy group antenatal care and childbirth education classes. *Journal of Perinatal Education*, 17(1): 27–34.

Walker, D., Visger, J. and Rossie, D. (2009) Contemporary childbirth education models. *Journal of Midwifery & Women's Health*, 54(6): 469–76.

Walsh, D. (1994) Management of progress in the first stage of labour. *Midwives Chronicle*, 107(1274): 84–8.

Walsh, D. (1997) *Evidence Based Care for Normal Labour and Birth*. London: Routledge.

Walsh, D. (1999) An ethnographic study of women's experience of partnership caseload midwifery practice: the professional as friend. *Midwifery*, 15(3): 165–76.

Walsh, D. (2005) Being inspired by childbirth activists. *Birthwrite, British Journal of Midwifery*, 13(5): 269.

Walsh, D. (2006a) 'Nesting' and 'matrescence': distinctive features of a free-standing birth centre. Available online in *Midwifery*, May 2006.

Walsh, D. (2006b) Subverting assembly-line birth: childbirth in a free-standing birth centre. *Social Science & Medicine*, 62(6): 1330–40.

Walsh, D. (2006c) Risk and normality in maternity care. In A. Symon (ed.) *Risk and Choice in Maternity Care*. London: Elsevier Science.

Walsh, D. (2007) A birth centre's encounters with discourses of childbirth: how resistance led to innovation. *Sociology of Health & Illness*, 29(2): 216–32.

Walsh, D. (2010) Childbirth embodiment: problematic aspects of current understandings. *Sociology of Health & Illness*, 32(3): 1–16.

Walsh, D. and Downe, S. (2004). Outcomes of free-standing, midwifery-led birth centres: a structured review of the evidence. *Birth*, 31(3): 222–9.

Walsh, D. and Newburn, M. (2002) Towards a social model of childbirth. Part 1. *British Journal of Midwifery*, 10(8): 476–81.

Walsh, D., Harris, M. and Shuttlewood, S. (1999) Changing midwifery birthing practice through audit. *British Journal of Midwifery*, 7(7): 432–5.

Walsh, T. (2009) Exploring the effects of hospital admission on contraction patterns and labour outcomes using women's perception of events. *Midwifery*, 25: 242–52.

Warren, C. (1999) Invaders of privacy. *Midwifery Matters*, 81: 8–9.

Waters, B. and Raisler, J. (2003) Ice water for the reduction of labour pain. *Journal of Midwifery & Women's Health*, 48: 317–21.

Wax, J., Lucas, F., Lamont, M., Pinette, M., Cartin, A. and Blackstone, J. (2010) Maternal and newborn outcomes in planned home birth vs planned hospital birth: a metasynthesis. *American Journal of Obstetrics & Gynecology*, 203: 1.e1–1.e8.

Wedin, K., Molin, J. and Crang Svalenius, E.L. (2008) Group antenatal care: new pedagogic method for antenatal care – a pilot study. *Midwifery*: doi:10.1016/j.midw.2008.10.010.

Wei, Shu-Qin, Luo, Zhong-Cheng, Xu, Hairong, Fraser, W.D. (2009) The effect of early oxytocin augmentation in labor: a meta-analysis. *Obstetrics & Gynecology*, 114(3): 641–9.

Wiberg-Itzel, E., Pettersson, H., Cnattingius, S. and Nordström, L. (2008) Association between lactate concentration in amniotic fluid and dysfunctional labor. *Acta Obstetrica et Gynaecologica*, 87(9): 924–8.

Wickham, S. (1999) Evidence-informed midwifery 1. *Midwifery Today*, Autumn 51: 42–3.

Wickham, S. (1999) Further thoughts on the third stage. *The Practising Midwife*, 2(10): 14–15.

Wiklund, I., Uvnas-Moberg, K., Ransjo-Arvidson, A. and Andolf, E. (2009) Epidural analgesia: breast-feeding success and related factors. *Midwifery*, 25: e31–e38.

Williams, A. (2003) Third-degree perineal tears: risk factors and outcome after primary repair. *Journal of Obstetrics & Gynaecology*, 23(6): 611–14.

Williams, A., Herron-Marx, S. and Hicks, C. (2007) The prevalence of enduring postnatal perineal morbidity and its relationship to perineal trauma. *Midwifery*, 23: 392–403.

Williams, K. and Galerneau, F. (2002) Fetal heart rate parameters predictive of neonatal outcome in the presence of a prolonged deceleration. *Obstetrics & Gynecology*, 100: 951–4.

Williams, M. and Chames, M. (2006) Risk factors for the breakdown of perineal laceration repair after vaginal delivery. *American Journal of Obstetrics & Gynecology*, 195: 755–9.

Winter, C. and Cameron, J. (2006) The 'stages' model of labour: deconstructing the myth. *British Journal of Midwifery*, 14(8): 454–7.

Winter, C. and Duff, M. (2010) The progress of labour: orderly chaos. In C. McCourt (ed.) *Childbirth, Midwifery and Concepts of Time*. London: Berghahn Books.

Winter, C., Macfarlane, A., Deneux-Tharaux, C. and Zhang, W. (2007) Variations in policies for management of the third stage of labour and the immediate management of postpartum haemorrhage in Europe. *BJOG*, 114: 845–54.

Witham-Leitch, M., Shelton, J. and Fleming, E., (2006) Central fetal monitoring: effect on perinatal outcomes and cesarean section rate. *Birth*, 33(4): 284–8.

Woods, T. (2006) The transitional stage of labour. *Midirs*, 16(2): 225–8.

World Health Organisation (1994) World Health Organisation partograph in management of labour. *Lancet*, 343(8910): 1399–404.

World Health Organisation (1997) *Care in Normal Birth: A Practical Guide*. Geneva: WHO.

Yancey, M., Zhang, J., Schwarz, J. *et al.* (2001) Labour epidural analgesia and intrapartum maternal hyperthermia. *Obstetrics & Gynecology*, 98(5): 763–70.

Yang, L., Chin, Y., Chen, W. and Wu, S. (1987) The effects of EMG biofeedback and autogenic training in relieving the anxiety of pregnant women. *Acta Psychologica Sinica*, 4: 420–5.

Yates, S. (2003) *Shiatsu for Midwives*. London: Books for Midwives Press.

Yelland, S. (2005) *Acupuncture in Midwifery*. London: Blackwell Publishing.

Yerby, M. (ed.) (2000) *Pain in Childbearing: Key Issues in Management*. London, Bailliere Tindall.

Yildirim, G. and Beji, N. (2008) Effects of pushing techniques in birth on mother and fetus: a randomized study. *Birth*, 35(1): 25–30.

Yildirim, G. and Sahin, N. (2004) The effect of breathing and skin stimulation techniques on labour pain perception of Turkish women. *Pain Research Management*, 9(4): 181–2.

Zadoroznyi, M. (1999) Social class, social selves and social control in childbirth. *Sociology of Health & Illness*, 21(3): 267–89.

Zain, H., Wright, J., Parrish, G. *et al.* (1998) Interpreting the fetal heart rate tracing: effects of knowledge of the neonatal outcome. *Journal of Reproductive Medicine*, 43: 367–70.

Zanetti-Dällenbach, R., Lapaire, O. and Maertens, A. (2006) Water birth, more than a trendy alternative: a prospective, observational study. *Archives of Gynecology and Obstetrics*, 274: 355–65.

Zhang, J., Landy, H. and Branch, W. (2010b) Contemporary patterns of spontaneous labor with normal neonatal outcomes. *Obstetrics & Gynecology*, 116(6): 1281–7.

Zhang, J., Troendle, J., Mikolajczyk, R. and Sundaram, R. (2010a) The natural history of the normal first stage of labour. *Obstetrics & Gynecology*, 115(4): 705–10.

Zhang, J., Troendle, J. and Yancey, M. (2002) Reassessing the labour curve. *American Journal of Obstetrics & Gynecology*. 187: 824–8.

Zwarenstein, M., Goldman, J. and Reeves, S. (2009) Interprofessional collaboration: effects of practice-based interventions on professional practice and healthcare outcomes. *Cochrane Database of Systematic Reviews*, Issue 3.

Zwarenstein, M., Stephenson, B. and Johnston, L. (2006) Case management: effects on professional practice and health care outcomes (Protocol). *Cochrane Database of Systematic Reviews*, Issue 3.

# Index